Chiropractic

AMAZING, ISN'T IT?

Dr. Claude Lessard
© 2003, 2012, 2019

I dedicate this book
to my children, Tara, Jeremy and Sabrina,
who are constant reminders that
Chiropractic is truly amazing.

Additional Titles

Chiropractic Amazing, Isn't It?

Quiropraxia ¿No Es Asombrosa?

La Chiropractique Incroyable N'est-ce pas?

Chiropractic Amazing, Isn't It? Workbook

Quiropraxia ¿No Es Asombrosa? Manual de Trabajo

A New Look at Chiropractic's Basic Science

Una Nueva Mirada a la Ciencia Básica de la Quiropráctica

TABLE OF CONTENTS

ACKNOWLEDGMENTS

The parts of a book, the words, sentences, paragraphs and pages seem to be the efforts of a single person. Only one name is credited as the author. This book however, is a collaboration of many individuals.

A humble thank you to all the patients, clients, and members who have put their confidence in our office. People who have had the courage to challenge me during the course of my career as an objective straight chiropractor.

Thank you to Dr. Thomas Gelardi, who had the vision to start Sherman College. A special thank you to Reggie, who gave me a philosophical ground. Thank you to my son, Jeremy, for the countless revisions, to my daughter Sabrina, and her friend, Doug, for the artwork, to my daughter Tara, for whom I work.

A special thank you to Christie Walther for her patience and for her honest opinion regarding much of this book. Special thanks to Tara for proofreading, Amanda Janiec for editing, and Jenny Troester Williams at Dreamwalker Productions for her help in making this second edition possible.

Thank you Jeanne D'Arc and Wellie Lessard for having imparted in me the love of work and la joie de vivre.

Finally, thank you to Sara for putting up with my peculiarities, for believing in me, for being my inspiration and for showing me that we cannot harvest what we do not sow, and we cannot sow where we are afraid to plow.

Dr. Claude Lessard

FOREWORD

A VISION OF HEALING

Dr. Claude Lessard has looked negativism squarely in the eye and thrown it from here to the St. Lawrence River. Now a successful chiropractor at 210 Makefield Road, Morrisville, PA, devoting his life to helping others, Lessard recalls his own youthful struggles as an undauntable "rebel" from Canada.

"When I was growing up," Lessard said, "I had different ideas." My parents would always remind me that my dreams were "unrealistic and impossible. That really frustrated me," he said. Maybe that is why Lessard devotes so much of his time to helping people deprogram negative principles. "We have been programmed by a culture very stiff in terms of do's and don'ts," he said, "and emerge as adults with excess negative baggage."

Lessard's hard work, insight, and "different" approach to mental and physical health have earned him the respect, admiration, and affection of his patients. He displays a book in his office filled with letters from satisfied patients, thanking him with heartfelt sincerity for relieving their pain and enhancing their lives.

Quebec, Canada is his birthplace, and the little village of Sainte Anne de Beaupre, with its bank along the St. Lawrence River, his hometown. "As a child," he said, "I would sit on top of the hill, look out over the mighty river, and dream, 'one day I am going to be in New York City.'"

Lessard met with plenty of hard work and opposition along the way to achieving his goals. "I dropped out of school in my senior year," he said, "and went to work at the papermill in Quebec for 522 days of hell." Lessard's job at the papermill was to clean up the residue from one of the sulfite treatment plants. "On the 522nd day," he continued, "I went down in the pit of the basement. It was dark, wet, hot, and noisy. The stench from the residue was everywhere, when a big thing happened. The handle on the wheelbarrow I was pushing broke. I sat down, looked around me, and knew I had had enough." His foreman had "the greatest belly laugh," he said, "when I told him I was leaving to go back to school, become a prominent doctor, and go to New York."

"When I first meet a patient," Lessard said, "I'm not meeting one individual. I am meeting a countless number of individuals" who have been influential in the patient's life. With a keen memory of his own struggles in pursuing his dream, Lessard is particularly sensitive to the individual needs of others. He does what he calls "deprogramming... to help people choose what is life promoting, rather than death promoting."

For Lessard, quitting his job and returning to school was only the beginning. "I did not speak English," he said, and for three months he studied English at night while finishing his high school education in the daytime. Lessard volunteered his time for two summers at the St. Anne's Shrine in Quebec for the opportunity to help people and speak English to religious pilgrims who came to witness miracles or receive divine healing.

On July 21, 1970, a group of pilgrims and six volunteer aides arrived at St. Anne's from New York City. It was on this day "I encountered Sara, my wife," he said, "she was a volunteer aide accompanying the group. We liked each other and by October I was enrolled at St. John's University in Jamaica, New York, as a pre-med student."

Life was not easy in New York as a student earning his way.

While in college, he made money cleaning cockroach infested apartments in Manhattan. "It was a hard, dirty job," he said, "but better than the pit at the papermill." He later found a "terrific" job in a circus called Adventures Inn. "I still have the tag that says 'The Gorilla Show,'" he said, "I was the gorilla."

Although Lessard reached his goal of going to New York City to study medicine, St. John's did not satisfy him in terms of healing techniques. He was continually disturbed about the side effects of medication and asked his toxicology professor, "Why are we using these drugs if their side effects are so well documented?" The teacher replied that the benefits outweighed the risks. When Lessard disagreed, the teacher questioned his aptness for the class. "At that point, I quit the University," he said.

That day, while walking down Broadway, Lessard met a friend, Jean-Claude Boucher, a chiropractic student from his hometown in Quebec. Within two hours, Boucher had completely sold Lessard on chiropractic care as a natural way of healing. "I was ready for this," he said, the idea of "promoting wellness rather than treating disease." Thereafter, he and his wife, Sara, and their daughter Tara, moved to South Carolina where Lessard attended Sherman College of Straight Chiropractic.

Those times were also challenging. "I went to school from 7 a.m. to 3 p.m. and worked at a gas station from 4 to 11 p.m. By 11:30, I was having dinner with my family," he said. "I studied until 3 a.m. and got up at 6 a.m. to do it all over again. Weekends he worked twelve hours a day, Saturday and Sunday.

After graduation in 1977, Lessard put his principles to task and opened his first practice on South Main Street in Yardley, PA. He was an instant success, and in 1983, moved his office's to his present location on Makefield Road.

He is co-founder of the Adio Institute of Straight Chiropractic in Horsham, PA, and is a member of the Masters, an elite group of 75 high achievers in the field of chiropractic. Lessard is the recipient of the Clinical Excellence and Philosophy Distinction Awards from Sherman College and won the 1991 Chiropractor of the Year Award from Markson Management Services, a chiropractic consulting firm in New York.

Lessard has turned the act of helping people into an art he passionately and sincerely cultivates. In 1985, he enrolled in a church ministry program of the Archdiocese of Philadelphia, to enhance his compassion skills, and graduated in 1987. Some of the benefactors have been Prevention for Abused Children of Bucks County, Catholic Charity Services, Bucks County Homeless, and the Interfaith Housing Corp.

"The most enjoyable part of my life today," he says, " is being an important part of people's lives. That's when I experience joy. That's when I enjoy life to the fullest."

Lessard lives in Yardley with his wife, Sara. Although he has reached unquestionable excellence in his profession, this dedicated healer says, "success is a journey that never ends but always challenges."

Sheree Birkbeck

INTRODUCTION

Maybe you are a seasoned, "veteran" chiropractic patient or doctor about to begin this book.

Or maybe you think "chiropractic" is the word the old guy behind the deli counter screams at you when you change your order for the third time in five minutes.

Regardless of the category you fall into, Dr. Claude Lessard energetically and passionately explains the art, science and philosophy of chiropractic in such a way that everyone, from doctors to first-time patients, can understand and become as excited about chiropractic as Claude! (Yes, it actually <u>is</u> possible!)

In this day and age, everyone is looking for the "magical" solution that will allow them to feel great and be happy. It's amazing that the ability for both of these to occur lies <u>within our own bodies</u>, just waiting to be released - as if the body were saying, "Hey! Let ME help YOU for once!"

As you turn each page, you too will be amazed by the incredible potential that your own body possesses to be healthy, happy, and full of abundant life! Claude has put his heart and soul into every enthusiastic page, with the hope that you will understand exactly why chiropractic is so important in attaining and maintaining true health and wellness, from infancy all the way through your "golden years." Claude will explain how your body can utilize every little bit of its own power to keep you healthy and feeling absolutely FANTASTIC, all the time! Best of all, you will learn that when you are healthy and feel terrific, you become stronger and more at peace mentally, which is that "magical" combination that people are looking for!

Search no more! That combination, as you will soon read, is what chiropractic is all about!

PREPARE TO BE AMAZED!

Jeremy Lessard

A LITTLE HISTORY

Five thousand years ago, Hypocrates stated: "One or more vertebrae of the spine may or may not go out of place very much. They might give way very little, and, if they do, they are likely to produce serious complications and even death, if not properly adjusted." History reveals that this statement by Hypocrates was totally ignored until 1895.

In Davenport, Iowa on September 18th of that year, Dr. Daniel David Palmer was trying to help his janitor, Harvey Lillard. Lillard had been deaf for 17 years as a result of hitting his head under a staircase and having felt something give in the lower part of his neck.

Dr. Palmer was examining the man and noticed a slight bump of his spine. Looking at his anatomy chart, Dr. Palmer concluded that one of the vertebrae was out of alignment and placed Lillard face down on a bench.

Dr. Palmer then, put his hands over the displaced vertebrae and gave it a quick short push not once, not twice, but three times. The third time he heard a "click" and Harvey Lillard could hear the noise made by the trolleys outside the buildings.

Of course, Dr. Palmer thought he had found the cure for deafness. So, he began advertising in the newspaper his new discovery. Many deaf people reportedly made appointments with Dr. Palmer. He adjusted them all. Some of them experienced significant improvements in their hearing, others not. However, still a certain number of people noted improvements in other areas of their health. Some improved their blood pressure, digestion, elimination and many more functions.

People with all kinds of conditions, began visiting Dr. Palmer and that's how the profession of chiropractic came to be. The name chiropractic came from the word chiros meaning hands and praktos meaning practice.

Chiropractic, whose time has arrived, is a humanitarian approach in caring for the human body.

NOTE TO THE READER

Over the last 45 years, many questions have often been asked of Straight Chiropractors in general of health related interests, specifically: natural health care, wellness programs and preventive maintenance.

I have written this book in a dialogue format questions and answers. Many questions deal with health related issues. However, with health being only 15% of the entire human experience, this book covers more than health. It relates most importantly to all physical activities, because human performance occurs as a result of body chemistry. There is not one single physical activity that does not depend on a change in your body chemistry somehow.

Therefore, in our lives, to whom do we turn for answers regarding life and health? Do we look to the massive computer of Douglas Adam's "Hitchhiker's Guide To The Galaxy," designed to give the ultimate answer that would completely explain all of life? If you read Adam's book, you realize that the computer takes almost eight million years to give the absolute answer and by the time the computer does this, everybody has forgotten the question. Do we look to medicine? Religion? Science? Psychology? Psychic hotlines? Astrology? To whom do we turn to?

Chiropractic is an art and a science developed from a philosophy which states that "Life and Health come from ABOVE-DOWN-INSIDEOUT", that there is an organization within this universe which is run by Intelligent Actions far greater than a super computer created by human beings. Chiropractic is based on deductive reasoning which begins with a major premise: "There is a Universal Intelligence in all matter constantly giving to it all of its properties and activities, thereby maintaining it in existence."

The first chapters explore the philosophy of chiropractic from a practical standpoint. Where do we come from? What makes us move, breathe and have our being? How do we function? How do we achieve our potential? Are we under the influence of an inner wisdom? Does it really matter?

The middle chapters deal with the emergence of scientific knowledge and follow the evolution of conscious information from the human brain to the human cell and from the human cell to the human brain. What is the major interference to the human body? What is the cause of malfunction? What is needed for the restoration of normal communication? Is it repeatable?

We will then look to the integrity of the Central Nerve System, its role and how it might indeed be related to the creative current of energy in matter, in mind and in human life.

The last chapters deal with the artistic and practical implication of a NEW system of healing using a NEW approach which relies on a NEW understanding and re-NEWed trust in the intelligence within all of us. However, our stance might be one of awe and simple application of a unique principle as we unfold toward our creative freedom and awareness. There might be answers and insights to this after all.

CLAUDE LESSARD, D.C.

PHILOSOPHY

WHAT IS A STRAIGHT CHIROPRACTOR?

A Straight Chiropractor is a Doctor of Chiropractic who understands the principles of chiropractic and uses them to help people better express their innate potential. The Straight Chiropractor is aware that all bodily functions are under the perfect control of the innate intelligence which uses the nerve system as means of communication.

The Straight Chiropractor knows the cause of interference to the communication system within the human body; it is called a vertebral subluxation. When there is a breakdown in communication, it alters the performance of the body decreasing its ability to reach its full innate potential. Therefore, the Straight Chiropractor locates, analyzes and corrects vertebral subluxations exclusively which are always causing a major interference to the nerve system disrupting communications resulting in improper function of the body. Once the vertebral subluxations are corrected, the life-force is restored insuring proper functions which allow the individuals to express more of their innate potential.

Any chiropractic practitioner doing something less than that, more than that, something different than that or for a different purpose than the one stated above, is not a Straight Chiropractor.

COULD YOU EXPLAIN WHAT INNATE INTELLIGENCE IS?

A simple understanding of our coming into existence will help us answer this great question.

You were conceived within the womb of your mother from two tiny cells: the sperm and the egg. They united and multiplied in nine months to a grand total of 400 trillion cells. A human baby at birth has a brain, a nerve system, a respiratory system, a circulatory system and many more systems, some of which are not yet known to science.

As you can see, your body is very well organized. The question to ask ourselves is: what causes organization? And the answer is: intelligent action causes organization!

Can you conceive of a complicated computer chip happening by sheer luck? Or a musical symphony composed by pure chance? Of course not! Evidently their fantastic organizations prove it takes intelligent individuals to create these complex systems.

Now do you think it possible that the creation of a human baby with all of its intricate internal systems happens by luck? Seriously the seven billion people populating our planet with similarly organized bodies are not haphazard occurrences Since your body is well organized, it must, logically speaking, be the result of an intelligence smart enough to assemble and organize it in the first place.

The organization of your body is under the perfect control of a great wisdom we call innate intelligence. Innate meaning "inborn, within you."

Everyone has an innate intelligence and no one can willingly control it. Suppose you had a pretzel for a snack. Just how much water would you have to drink to neutralize the salt? How much faster must your heart beat, should you run to catch a bus, chop some firewood or do any kind of exercise? How much sugar must be burned within your body in order to maintain it at 98.6 degrees of human temperature?

Well, now, these questions need not bother you a bit. There is not a chemist or a scientist in the world who can tell you. But that liver of yours can handle the sugar problem if you never even saw the inside of a textbook of chemistry. Your heart, the number of heartbeats and the stomach will call for its water and tell you when it gets enough. Your innate intelligence uses your nerve system to communicate and control every function of every system, organ, gland and cell known and unknown within your body.

AMAZING ISN'T IT?

HOW CAN THE BODY NOT PERFORM PROPERLY?

Since your innate intelligence coordinates ALL of your body functions through your nerve system, it is very important that your nerves be free of any obstruction or interference caused by a vertebral subluxation. Because, like fiber optic wires, if the nerves are cut off or if they are obstructed or otherwise disturbed, the particular organ or area which those nerves serve will alter its functions. It is like a camcorder, in perfect working order but with no battery power, nothing to make it record. In order for your body to perform properly, it must be working right. Your life-force must flow through your nerves uninterrupted to every system, organ, gland and cell of your body.

Let us remember that whenever one of your nerves is disturbed, some part of your body cannot receive the life-force sent by your INNATE INTELLIGENCE and your body will not perform properly, depending on the extent of the interference. If this interference is caused by a vertebral subluxation and is corrected, normal function is reestablished, giving once again perfect control to your innate intelligence allowing your body to receive complete life-force and perform exactly as it was intended.

AMAZING ISN'T IT?

WHAT EXACTLY IS VERTEBRAL SUBLUXATION?

The human body functions as a chemical factory as well as an electric power plant. It is under the perfect control of the innate intelligence of the body which uses the nerve system to send chemo-electrical impulses to communicate with all the cells of that body. Those impulses have only one purpose: to allow the body to function properly. If the life-force which is encoded within those impulses leaving the brain and coursing through the nerve system is received precisely as it was intended by the innate intelligence, the systems, organs, glands and all the cells of the body will be performing efficiently. The result of such performance is a greater expression of the innate potential of the body.

The innate potential relates to the entire human experience. Since the nerve system carries the life-force throughout the body, it is very well protected. A structure of bones called the vertebral column surrounds the nerve system.

The vertebral column is held in place by the back muscles and ligaments. This column of bone is rather flexible to allow a multitude of movements. However, because of its flexibility, some of the segments of the vertebral column called vertebrae may go out of alignment and in doing so, put pressure on the delicate nerves exiting between those vertebrae. This is called: vertebral subluxation.

A vertebral subluxation always results in altering the flow of the life-force encoded within the chemo-electric impulses coursing within the nerve system, thus causing the body to malfunction.

If the body is not working right, its performance will diminish affecting all the systems within that body. The immune system will function improperly, the resistance of the body will decrease, other systems will be impaired, the repairing and healing mechanisms will be inefficient which will allow the cells to lose their ability to excrete properly, to be productive and to reproduce themselves normally. In short, the entire body will, over time, re-create itself abnormally.

The person may not feel bad, have symptoms or pain immediately, but if the body is not working right for weeks, months or years, the expression of its innate potential will diminish and the entire human experience of the person will be affected.

Most of the time, vertebral subluxations do not hurt and this is why everyone needs their vertebral column checked for the detection of vertebral subluxations. Straight Chiropractors are trained to locate, analyze and correct vertebral subluxations. If one or more vertebral subluxations are detected, they will perform a specific adjustment. If they do not find any subluxations, they will see the person at their next appointment for another check-up.

AMAZING ISN'T IT?

LUXURY OR NEED?

"I have been under chiropractic care and my friends have noticed my health improvement... yet, when I tell them chiropractic care is good for them, too, they reply that there is nothing wrong with their backs. What should I tell them?"

This question is quite pertinent, as this attitude is extremely common in our society. I believe the first thing people have to realize is the fact that vertebral subluxations (small displacements of a spinal bone) almost always goes unnoticed. Generally there are no apparent changes, discomfort, pain or lack of motion in the spine. Yet dysfunction, dis-coordination, lack of proper control between the brain (the master controller of all human function) and the rest of the body exists for most of us since the moment of birth! It is a matter of fact since almost everyone born in a hospital through the so-called "normal birth process" is born with a vertebral subluxation located in the neck or lower back. Most people do not notice it, for they have nothing to compare it to!

According to Dr. Chuang Suh, head of the department of spinal biomechanics at the University of Colorado, 95% of children under the age of five have one or more vertebral subluxations and 100% of those over five years of age have one or more vertebral subluxations. In other words, this situation is indigenous to our modern society.

Your friends must become aware that as soon as the baby's head came out of it's mother's womb, someone came along to "help Nature" and grabbed that baby's head, twisted it and turned it around to induce a torsion of the cervical spine (neck) in order to force the shoulders to turn and pass longitudinally through the birth canal. This routine procedure causes vertebral subluxation almost 100% of the time.

Now a vertebral subluxation does not produce immediate symptoms, pain or death, just a progressively slow decrease of vital energy flow between the brain and the rest of the body. Given time it will always diminish the innate potential of that body, produce malfunction, symptoms, disease and death.

Straight Chiropractors are vitally concerned and interested in correcting vertebral subluxations, thus removing interference to the nerve system. This in turn, allows you to function at your optimum innate potential so that you may reach a stage of physical, mental and social well-being. You cannot touch one without touching the others.

Nature needs no help, just no interference! Life, health, and your right to an exciting, intense and happy existence were taken away from you at your very birth. It is time now to regain it, for after all, it is your God-given birthright!

AMAZING ISN'T IT?

SICK AND TIRED OF BEING SICK AND TIRED?

Chiropractic works because it allows that permanent law of life within to be released and to manifest itself without interference.

As a Straight Chiropractor, one of the best ways I can explain chiropractic is to turn to the outside world and examine what we see at work in nature. After all, isn't everything outward also inward?

From the movement and balance of our internal body water (intercellular and intracellular fluids), from the hatching of a baby chick to the natural process of birth in humans, from the awakening of plants and animals at sunrise to the awakening of a child in the morning... similarities abound so let us compare your body to a beautiful garden.

The brain is the well producing life-sustaining water; the brain stem is the faucet; the spinal cord is the main pipeline carrying the water to the garden; the nerves are the main water hoses going to various organs of your body; the sprinklers are the millions of nerve fibers watering every single cell of your body. The innateintelligence of your body is the Gardener.

Now, as long as the quantity of water determined by the Gardener can flow freely through the main pipeline toward the various and numerous hoses and sprinklers, the garden can be watered and Life can be expressed to its fullest and so provide a more complete human experience, 15% of which happens to be health.

If we were to interfere with the natural flow of water by turning down the faucet or putting a stone on the main pipeline or any of the many hoses, the water flow would decrease to some extent and the sprinklers would spin slower, not spraying water as far or as well as it was intended by the Gardener.

Given some time, (for there is no process that does not require time), some plants, or fruits, or vegetables would weaken (fatigue), others would change colors (symptoms), others would change sizes (more symptoms), while still others would grow wild (inflammation, infection, tumors), some would become rotten (degeneration), and eventually, some would die (organ failures).

Traditionally and conventionally the sickness-curers and disease-treaters walk through the garden of your body, look around, test this plant, that flower, this fruit or vegetable and from this outside-in approach and they make-up a diagnosis. Then, they proceed to treat and prognosticate whatever they think is going wrong. "See that plant over there, it looks weak, let's give it an injection to stimulate it. Those fruits there are getting out of hand, let's prescribe pills to inhibit them. See these vegetables, they're too pale, let's cover them with oils to make them shiny. Now, the flowers by the fence are wilting, let's chop them down. And this shrub right here is too ugly, let's replace it with an artificial one. And finally, all those little patches of brown grass, let's kill them by using antibiotic chemicals."

Please, tell me what kind of care has been applied to the garden of your body? Your body still looks very good, but unfortunately, it only looks good. It is doing much worse than before because some parts are missing, and the water is still not flowing freely to feed the roots. And also, help me understand what would happen to a healthy body if we were to give it drugs every day? Would it not eventually get sick? Therefore, explain to me if drugs given to a healthy body make it sick, how is it possible for a sick body to get well if we give it drugs? No one yet has given me an answer to this question.

The Straight Chiropractor understands chiropractic philosophy which states that there is an innate intelligence within the body that is in perfect control of all its parts providing there is no interference with its natural flow of energy. Therefore, turn up the faucet or remove the stones causing pressure on the hoses, let the water flow, allow the garden to be watered, and given time, life will return to the garden... from within.

Chiropractic does not address the symptoms, pain or feelings because they are results of a cause. When cells are sick, they never recover, they always die just the same as healthy cells die every second of your life. Of course they are replaced by new cells, and if the new cells are as sick as the ones that just died, the person is as sick as before. If the new cells are sicker than the ones that just died, the person is getting worse. And if the new cells are healthier than the ones that just died, then the person is getting better.

Do you think that the parts of the garden lacking the right amount of water will replace themselves normally or abnormally? How about if the water supplied by the pipelines of the garden would be restored to its natural flow to all the flowers, plants, fruits, vegetables and shrubs, would they replace themselves normally or abnormally compared to the ones without the proper flow? Chiropractic philosophy states: A vertebral subluxation which is an interference to the flow of mental impulses from the brain to the cells of the body always causes a decreased expression of innate potential, thereby promoting malfunction within the body. Chiropractic philosophy also states: Correct the vertebral subluxation and it will restore the flow of mental impulses from the brain to the cells of the body and will always cause an increased expression of innate potential, thereby improving function within the body.

AMAZING ISN'T IT?

WHERE ARE YOU? SOMEWHERE-IN-BETWEEN?

1. When nerves are cut-off. LIFE is cut-off.
2. When LIFE is cut-off, the result is death.

Chiropractic is not a treatment or a therapy for any disease condition. The purpose of chiropractic is to facilitate a better expression of life within the body.

1. Wholeness or health = Total life.
2. Death = Total absence of life.
3. Somewhere-in-between = Partial life.

When Life is choked off to any extent, we have a situation called partial (partial life, partial ease [dis-ease], partial function, partial control, partial coordination, etc.). Even if people feel well, when some of their life is choked off, they are not at a stage of wholeness or health (ease), so consequently they are at the stage of DIS-EASE (partial everything).

At the stage of dis-ease the body progresses to such an extent that many tissue cells malfunction and break down. Signs, symptoms and even pain will eventually appear. The person has a disease when these symptoms manifest themselves within the body.

It may take a person as long as four to six years before symptoms appear (like cancer, kidney stones, and arthritis for example). As you know, these diseases do not develop overnight. Why sit around waiting for symptoms to develop? The hospitals are filled with people who just last week had no signs or symptoms and now they are dying.

The famous philosopher Aldous Huxley once said: "Facts do not cease to exist because they are ignored."

AMAZING ISN'T IT?

IS IT AS SIMPLE AS THAT?

The human body is a powerhouse of LIFE and ENERGY. The innate intelligence of the body is the master controller of everything known and unknown about you. Innate intelligence uses your brain as the generator of life-energy, the spinal cord as the main high-tension wire between the brain and the body, and the nerves as secondary wires running from the spinal cord to the organs, glands and every other part of the body.

The spinal cord is sheathed in a protective tube called the vertebral column. In order to allow freedom of movement, the vertebral column is flexible in all directions. It is composed of 24 movable segments called vertebrae. The structure of the vertebrae is one of the most complex bone structures of the entire body. The joints between the vertebrae is the most complex joints of the entire body.

When the spinal cord or spinal nerves have pressure exerted on them by displacements of one or more vertebrae, called vertebral subluxations, normal communication between the brain and the rest of the body is altered. The innate expression of that body is diminished and trouble begins, unnoticed at first. Given time, the tissue cells involved in the altered communication begin to lose their ability to be productive, lose their ability to excrete properly and lose their ability to reproduce themselves normally. Eventually signs and symptoms will appear, first mildly and sooner or later the organs, glands or systems involved break down. Then as this gets most people's attention, it leads them to seek help.

On the other hand, when the spinal cord or spinal nerves are free from interference caused by vertebral subluxations, the innate intelligence of the body is using the brain to communicate normally and precisely with the cells of the body. This allows the cells to be productive, excrete properly and reproduce themselves normally. The result is a body functioning correctly at all times, performing at its best and expressing more of its innate potential. The entire human experience is enhanced and health (being 15% of the human experience) is improved. The rest of the human experience, spiritual life, family life, work life, social life, financial life, etc... functions with efficiency.

Chiropractic has only one goal: to locate, analyze and correct vertebral subluxations in accordance with its philosophy. This allows every man, woman and child to express more of their innate potential. The end result is a true state of life expression, coordination, and human performance enhancing mental and intellectual abilities and more creativity.

The Straight Chiropractor is concerned in keeping your nerve system free of interference by searching for the presence of vertebral subluxations and correcting them. This is the KEY to true life expression and enjoyment. It is as simple as that!

AMAZING ISN'T IT?

NATURAL OR ARTIFICIAL?

Wouldn't it be wonderful to live in a world of freedom where we could breathe fresh air without the need of nasal spray? Wouldn't it be wonderful to walk barefoot in the grass without corn pads? Wouldn't it be wonderful to keep one's cool all day without the use of Prozac?

Wouldn't it be wonderful to walk with one's head held high without a neckbrace? Wouldn't it be wonderful to be happy-go-lucky without Valium? Wouldn't it be wonderful to be vibrant and strong at 70 without Metamucil #1 #2 #3 #4? Wouldn't it be wonderful to be ready for a good night's sleep without the aid of Sominex?

Wouldn't it be wonderful to live with all your organs and glands without fear of losing them through operations? Wouldn't it be wonderful to face life and every new day with a smile and much enthusiasm?

We have lived too long in the shadow of our own ignorance and fears. We should live in the land of bright sunlight, like a skylark. We must cleanse our body of nerve interference and allow ourselves to achieve more of our human potential. Under the care of a Straight Chiropractor, this can and would be accomplished. Then and only then can we improve the functions of our body by allowing the flow of mental impulse through our nerve system to be uninterrupted from above-down-inside-out. Perhaps a life in a world of coordination and peace begins with ourselves first.

Chiropractic is a method allowing the body to normally assert its own inherent natural functions. Are you familiar with the term "natural functions?" You know, the repairing, healing and restoring back to normal of the human body are natural functions. Some other natural functions of a normally functioning body are: complete reparation of wounds... successful healing and mending of fractures... proficiently warding off environmental germs... normalization of emotional strain... resisting invading foreign organisms...

If your natural functions are not up to par, if the various normal internal mechanisms involved are impaired or interfered with, then we recognize that you are not expressing your innate potential and that you are in a state of dis-ease (malfunction and incoordination) and may eventually, given time, develop signs, symptoms, pain and even an untimely death.

The Straight Chiropractor understands the principles of natural body functions and is concerned in locating, analyzing and correcting interferences to these natural body functions. These interferences are called: vertebral subluxations.

Chiropractic has built a philosophy, science and art around the correction of vertebral subluxations based on a definite set of principles (more than 30) to follow in order to achieve the understanding of the ultimate importance and priority of correcting vertebral subluxations. Straight Chiropractors concern themselves thoroughly and exclusively with the application of those principles.

By consistently and persistently checking the spines of people for the presence of vertebral subluxations and correcting them, the Straight Chiropractor helps people to express more of their innate potential and allows their natural functions to be normalized at the greatest and highest level of proficiency available today.

Wouldn't it be wonderful to learn to live in freedom and knowledge rather than in bondage and ignorance of what is truly good for us?

AMAZING ISN'T IT?

IS THIS THE TURNING POINT?

Health makes up approximately 15% of the human experience and it is our individual responsibility. If we desire to achieve our full potential, then we must do what is necessary and be willing to pay the price. First, we must know what true health is. Health is defined as a condition of wholeness in which all the organs and glands of the body are functioning 100% at all times.

This means that in order to be healthy we must have all of our organs and glands, and they must function properly all the time. We now see that health and function are inter-related and dependent on one another. Next we need to know what controls the functions in the body and where it comes from.

Gray's Anatomy, a textbook recognized world-wide within the scientific community states that the purpose of the brain and the nerve system is to control and coordinate the functions of the other tissues, organs and glands of the body and to relate the body to its environments both internal and external.

Straight Chiropractors understand that the innate intelligence of the body is what controls and coordinates the functions of the body by using the brain and nerve system as its means of communication. We see, perhaps for the first time, that the responsibility for proper body functions lies not with drugs, needles, surgeries and radiations, but with the innate intelligence of the body perfectly controlling the functions of the body. Simply stated, this means that if your brain and nerve system are working properly, allowing all parts of your body to function 100% all the time, you will be truly healthy.

Vertebral subluxations are interferences to the natural flow of mental impulses from the brain through the nerve system to all the parts of the body, which cause your body to function less than 100% and achieve less than your normal potential, therefore enjoying less health.

Straight Chiropractors search for the presence of vertebral subluxations in people's vertebral columns. When they are located, analyzed and corrected, this allows the body to function once again at 100%, thereby increasing your ability to express more of your innate potential and become healthier.

AMAZING ISN'T IT?

CAN ANYONE BUILD ONE HUMAN CELL OUT OF THE ELEMENTS OF NATURE?

Humankind has been studying the human body dead and alive, sick and well, in an organized manner for about 5,000 years. We have systematized, computerized, and stored all this mass of dead and alive information in countless data bases dividing it into multiple subjects. We have spewed all of this education through colleges, universities, libraries and the internet into billions of brains through thousands of years. We have deduced theories, tried them, discarded them and tried again. We have experimented and practiced our "education" on people for all kinds of reasons anywhere and everywhere in all kinds of cases.

If it were possible to condense all this information: discard all these premises, condense it all into an essence and inject it into the brain of one person, in one laboratory, there wouldn't be one university graduate who could manufacture, make, or synthesize ONE tissue cell, organize its elements, compound its ingredients, and cause it to live, to adapt and to reproduce itself.

Yet, within every woman, be she white, black, yellow or red; uneducated or college graduate, Asian, African, Aborigines or American, Jewish, Muslim, Christian, Buddhist or Atheist, there is an innate intelligence that can and does make 400 trillion tissue cells in two hundred eighty days.

Not only does innate intelligence make these cells, it organizes them into respective kinds to do certain types of work, properly distributes each into its respective locality and builds them into various organs to do various functions. The innate intelligence organizes each individual cell with every other single cell into one harmonious body, causes all cells to coordinate one tissue with another and one organ with another into systems, chemically, mechanically, electrically, magnetically and functionally. Then, at the proper time and place, it causes them to begin working, each with each other's parts.

In due time, the innate intelligence builds the structure so it reproduces its own kind.

Now if we could, how would we build a baby?

AMAZING ISN'T IT?

"DOCTOR, CAN YOU CURE ME, PLEASE?"

Throughout our day, we pick up bits and pieces of conversations emanating from our reception rooms. Often times we have heard people saying: "Chiropractic cured me from migraines, high blood pressure, paralysis, menstrual cramps and what not, from hyperfunction to hypofunction." Well, let's bring things back into focus.

Straight Chiropractors do not cure anything. Why? Simply because they cannot! Any healing of the human body is done by the innate intelligence of the body from within.

It is electricity which produces light, not the electrician turning on the switch... It is the steam which gives heat, not the plumber operating the valve... It is the software which computerizes information, not the computer operator... It is the water which grows the fruits, not the gardener opening the faucet... It is the energy within you which gives you life, grows you from baby to child, to adult. It is the energy within you which allows you to live... which, if interfered with, decreases the expression of your innate potential and causes your body to malfunction... which, when restored, increases the expression of your innate potential and causes your body to function normally.

AMAZING ISN'T IT?

NORMAL VS. ABNORMAL?

Remember that the difference between a corpse and a living body is the absence or presence of the life energy within those bodies.

The difference between normal expression of your innate potential and abnormal expression of your innate potential is the degree of integrity of your nerve system. One of the factors influencing the integrity of the nerve system is the normal or abnormal quantity and quality flow of the intangible life-energy within.

Vertebral Subluxations are interferences to the nerve system which result in the abnormal quantity and quality flow of the intangible life-energy within.

The Straight Chiropractor, by locating, analyzing and correcting vertebral subluxations, allows the body to once again regain integrity of its nerve system by regulating normal quantity and quality of the intangible life-energy within. Then the body has a greater chance to heal, due to a better expression of its innate potential.

AMAZING ISN'T IT?

"ARE WE ALL ALIKE OR ALL DIFFERENT?"

Society is often compared to anthills or beehives. It harbors human beings who seem to function like social insects, with huge numbers of them playing identical roles in the community and returning to their appointed cells morning and evening, as if they were but interchangeable units in a complex colony.

Scholars have contributed to this collective, anonymous view of humankind by emphasizing in their studies those attributes shared by all human beings. They have discovered generalizations which apply to biological man, social man, political man, economic man, man in the abstract. But in the real world, no two human beings are alike, and all prize their individuality above everything else. We seem to care little for universality because we cherish our uniqueness.

All members of the human species share the same fundamental anatomic structures, physiologic needs, and mental attributes, but the similarities go much further. Whatever the pigmentation of the skin and the thickness of the lips, a smile is a smile everywhere. The facial expression and behavioral patterns expressing love, anger, surprise, and fear are common to all.

Civilizations differ from period to period and from place to place, but they are all based on the same biological drives and fixed action patterns. Poems of love or sorrow and monuments celebrating worship or triumph are universally meaningful. A Chinese lullaby or one from a Western country will be just as soothing to either an Asian or American child. Cosmetics for heightening the lines of the eyes have been found in Neolithic remains and have been used in one form or another by all people at all times, as have masks, kingly robes, and decorative arts.

Irrespective of origin, people are much more alike than they are different. A good friend of mine, Fr. Curtis Clark put it this way: "We are uniquely the same" he says, and in spite of this uniformity we never forget that we differ in geographical and national backgrounds, in religious and philosophical allegiances, and most importantly in the mysterious combination of qualities and defects which makes each one of us a unique specimen of the human species.

Most scientific studies of the human development deal with human beings as if they were the passive product of genetic and environmental forces... biological robots. However, there is something within human beings which concerns itself with regulation and control of adaptation. This latter approach is justified by the fact that each child is born with a particular body and a particular nerve system, that each mother has her own style of motherhood which is the result of her own life in a given society at a given moment of history, and that surroundings affect all phases of development.

It is quite clear then, that what must happen to keep the body alive (the minimum supply necessary) and what must not happen, lest one die or be severely stunted (the maximum frustration and interference possible) is an increasing leeway in regard to what may happen. Obviously, a maximum nerve supply and minimum interference will help us better express our innate potential which will influence our human experience and our happenings. To this cause, the Straight Chiropractor is committed.

AMAZING, ISN'T IT?

HOW CAN WE PROTECT OURSELVES AGAINST DISEASE?
WHY BE AFRAID OF ANYTHING?

Watching television, you would think we live at bay, in total jeopardy, surrounded on all sides by enemies, human-seeking germs, shielded against infection and death only by a chemical technology that enables us to keep killing them off. We are instructed to spray disinfectants everywhere, into the air of our bedrooms and kitchens and with special energy into our bathrooms, since it is our very own germs that seem the worst kind.

We explode clouds of aerosol into our noses, mouths, underarms, and privileged crannies.

We apply potent antibiotics, creating antibiotic-resistant bacteria, to minor scratches and seal them with plastic. Plastic is the new protector: we wrap the already plastic tumblers of hotels in more plastic, seal the toilet seat like state secrets after irradiating them with ultraviolet light. We live in a world where the microbes are always trying to get at us, to tear us cell from cell, and we only stay alive and whole through diligence and fear.

Does this really make sense? We think of human diseases as the work of an organized, modernized kind of underground "bad guys" in which bacteria are the most visible and centrally placed of our adversaries. We assume that they must somehow relish what they do. Do they come after us for profit? And are there so many of them that diseases seem inevitable? A natural part of the human condition? Come on! These are paranoid delusions! This is pure belief in superstitions! Please, take just one moment to think about it.

In real life, even in our worst circumstances we have always been a relatively minor interest of the vast world of germs, bacteria, viruses and microbes. Diseases are not the rule. Indeed, it occurs so infrequently and involves such a relatively small number of species (considering the huge population of bacteria on the earth) that it has a freakish aspect. Diseases result from inconclusive negotiations within the body having a cause.

The same innate intelligence that is within you is also within every single living organism on this planet. Therefore, since the brain and the nerve system coordinate the negotiations with in the human organism, it certainly is common sense to have it function normally with no interference. The Straight Chiropractor is dedicated to maintaining the integrity of the human nerve system by locating, analyzing and correcting vertebral subluxations which are a major cause of interference to the nerve system, thereby affecting the negotiations of the human body with its environment.

When the body is functioning normally, it expresses more of its innate potential and negotiates accordingly.

AMAZING ISN'T IT?

"IS THERE A BUG GOING AROUND?"

In the 21st century, it is still a common belief that due to obscure events or bad luck "we catch a cold" or that "there is a bug going around."

This social programming never ceases to amaze me. In 1976 it was the "swine flu," 1981 the "Asian flu," 1987 the "Korean flu" and 1998 it was the "Bird flu" from Hong Kong... and who knows what the year 2025 will bring along... You don't "catch" a cold nor is the "bug going around" in the sense that the normally virus-free body suddenly becomes overwhelmed by a virulent horde of invading microbes.

Cold viruses are as ubiquitous as the air we breathe. They live in the healthy mouth, sinuses and throat tissues, which usually protect the body from viral attack. The tissues are covered with microscopic hairs called cilia and a thin blanket of mucus. The moist mucus traps the virus particle, like flypaper, and its mildly acidic chemical composition blocks their reproduction long enough for the cilia to sweep them into the stomach where powerful digestive acids kill them. The micro-ecology of the healthy throat also involves subtle interactions between body temperature and blood flow that reinforce the area's anti-viral mission.

Fatigue, stress, overworking, lack of sleep, anxiety and poor diet are all life factors that contribute to vertebral subluxation which in turn causes a change in normal nerve supply to the body. This condition upsets the delicate micro-ecology of the throat, leaving it dry, less acidic and a bit cooler. These changes allow virus particles to penetrate the mucus layers, invade throat cells and reproduce.

Curing a cold therefore, does not involve "eradicating cold germs," but rather restoring healthy tissue equilibrium that inhibit viral reproduction. Strange as it may seem, that is precisely what cold symptoms do.

Sore throat, runny nose, stuffy head and fever are the manifestation of the body's efforts to re-establish a healthy balance in the throat. The appearance of cold symptoms means that the body has deployed its healing forces.

Science News (November, 1996) reports that cold viruses respond to a chemical released by cancer cells within the human body attacking the cancer cells, and ingesting them. This basically means that to have a "cold" is good to fight cancer within human being. Studies done in Ukraine reveal that people having three to four "colds" per year have lesser chances of developing cancer. When cold viruses penetrate the mucus blanket, their reproduction kills cancer cells. As these cells die, they release several substances, one of which is called histamine. Histamines cause the tiny blood vessels, or capillaries, in the infected area to expand. Capillary expansion stimulates increased blood flow into the area. This increased blood volume carries with it white blood cells and antibodies that attack the virus.

As blood bathes the infected area, the throat becomes red and raw. Meanwhile, some of the fluid in the extra blood in the infected area drains out of the capillaries and into the "Nasopharynx," the area behind the mouth where the nose and throat join. This fluid mixes with mucus to produce the runny nose and stuffed-up feelings usually associated with colds. Fever increases metabolism and promotes healing by spurring the elimination of dead cells and the creation of new ones. Fever also heats the body temperature beyond the range for viral reproduction. All these incredible events are all under the direct control of the innate intelligence of the body using the nerve system to carry out its intent.

AMAZING ISN'T IT?

ARE WE WORKING OVERTIME?

All of you who have a "cold" every now and again, pay attention to what I am writing in this segment.

The symptoms of a cold do not result directly from the destruction of cells by viruses, but from the body's response to this destruction – specifically, the inflammation that accompanies the immune system's attack on the virus.

Therefore, anyone taking some type of medication trying to suppress or mask the symptoms of a cold, is in realit, fighting the necessary response of the immune system's attack on the virus. This means that the innate intelligence of the body must work "overtime" to kill the virus in addition to eliminate the drug one takes.

Let us understand, that under viral attack, cells in the mucus membranes of the nose release histamine, blood capillaries in the area dilate, and blood serum leaks into the tissues of the membrane. The membrane swells. Some of its tissues secrete more mucus, not all of which can easily move up through the constricted nasal passages. The excess simply runs out. An overload of mucus in the throat excites nerve endings that stimulate a cough, which clears the passage before the virus-laden mucus can move down into the lungs. The swelling and cell damage stimulates receptors in the nose, triggering a sneeze. Your head feels stuffy and congested, your nose runs, your throat is sore. Each sneeze and cough releases outside the body a spray of droplets loaded with virus particles in an attempt to heal the body from the cold.

AMAZING ISN'T IT?

WHAT IS THIS SOMETHING?

Life takes on new meaning when we wake up to that special something that lies in each one of us. That "something" is the faith and courage to pursue our individual talents and dreams, but it is more than this.

That "something," our silent partner through life, is an intelligence regulating all of our body activities without educated, conscious thought. This silent partner... inborn intelligence... converts our food from yesterday into flesh and blood today. That "something" is the mysterious system of the body that heals broken bones, cuts, scrapes and bruises.

In life terms, we should do all we can to assist our silent partner in body processes. If this innate intelligence is capable of healing broken bones, bruises and scrapes, then it should be capable of restoring other functions of the body. All our innate intelligence needs is proper access to the troubled parts of the body for healing to occur.

Chiropractic is based on assisting this process of that "something" within... our innate intelligence. When our innate intelligence is obstructed or hindered, then negotiation on the part of the body with its internal and external environments is impaired.

Chiropractic care is designed to locate, analyze and correct the interference called vertebral subluxation and allow the power of our innate intelligence within the body to be released for maximum restoration and to recover its normal balance.

The power to enjoy normal function... normally and simply... is accomplished by releasing the power of that "something" that commands all healing.

AMAZING ISN'T IT?

SCIENCE

WHAT IS BODY CHRONOLOGY?

Human growth proceeds in four phases. The first, before birth, results mainly from cell division. All nerve cells, for example, are present by the sixth month of pregnancy; the nerve system continues to grow as these cells enlarge. During the second phase, from birth to maturity, the enlargement of existing cells tends to dominate. A baby's heart contains the same number of cells as the larger organ. It grows only by enlargement. During the third phase, maturity, emphasis switches to the maintenance of existing functions and the repair of damage from injury or wear and tear. When old age, the final phase, sets in, slowed growth can no longer replace lost cells, and the efficiency of our organs and tissues decline.

All of the above mentioned phases are under direct control of the innate intelligence of the body. It is quite fascinating to witness the chronology of these phases within each and every one of us. It suffices to say that the innate intelligence of the body works miracles constantly. All we have to do is to be grateful by taking good care of our bodies.

AMAZING ISN'T IT?

DO WE HAVE CYCLES?

Did you ever notice that everything in life seems to go in cycles? To get down to basics, there's our life cycle: from infancy, childhood, adolescence, adulthood and old age. Well, researchers have found that most aspects of our lives do occur in cycles. The same is true for the working of our bodies. There are numerous cycles constantly repeating over and over an infinite number of times, and, there is one cycle in particular that chiropractic deals with. This is called "THE SIMPLE CYCLE". The simple cycle is a continuous cycle which actually begins and ends at the same point; and then again, it doesn't really end, does it? The brain is the creator of a mental image which is then transformed to energy and, by means of efferent nerves, the impulse comes out from the center and is transmitted to the periphery, or tissue cells. Once again, transmission will occur in the opposite direction from tissue cell to brain cell, and as you know this occurs via afferent nerves.

This is so important because it is the reason that our bodies are alive. It's the reason that our body has the ability to grow and heal itself. Chiropractic deals specifically with this philosophy. Don't be fooled and think that a chiropractor heals you. Only the body has the ability to heal itself. When an adjustment is given, the body is restored to its maximum ability to send chemoelectrical impulses to all of the organs, and then back to the brain. The cycle is meant to be continuous. Any interference in that cycle will affect the ability of the body to function properly.

AMAZING ISN'T IT?

HOW MUCH ARE YOU WORTH?

Some time back, an article was published which calculated the value of all the chemicals in the human body. At the going price, the final figure was somewhere around $0.98!! What they were saying is that the human body is really a combination of water (hydrogen and oxygen), carbon and such minerals as iron, potassium, sodium and numerous other elements. If the body were broken down into its simplest components, the market value would be less than a dollar. In one sense that tends to be quite humbling. However, as you think more about it, there are some pretty fantastic thoughts to be gained. It goes without saying that we place more value than a dollar on human life. Tell the parents that are looking into the face of a newborn that their little baby, because of its size is not even worth $0.98. The being part of a human being makes the value so high that it cannot be measured in dollars and cents.

But the $0.98 chemical value of a human is also a misleading figure. True, that may be the value of the body in its simplest state but a body does not exist that way. Blood is made up of potassium, sodium, hydrogen, etc. However, the eight pints or so in your body are highly valued. Interferon is a substance your body produces from the above elements. Scientists are just now beginning to produce it commercially for the treatment of disease at a cost of millions of dollars per ounce! Any diabetic will tell you of the expense of a days supply of insulin which is not even human insulin. Can you imagine the value of insulin produced in exactly the right human quality for your particular body and in the right amount? Adrenalin, cortisone, and all other hormones are nothing but carbon, hydrogen, and oxygen and all those other elements valued at $0.98. What is it then that increases their value so greatly? It is the inborn wisdom of your body which is able to transform that $0.98 worth of substances into chemical compounds, and fluids worth millions of dollars. It is this same wisdom which every day in and day out organizes every cell in the body and keeps your body working as it was intended.

AMAZING ISN'T IT?

DO YOU KNOW YOUR CIRCULATORY SYSTEM IS THE RIVER OF LIFE?

Within the human body flows a river unlike any other earthly river – a crimson stream that courses through every organ, twists past every cell on a journey that stretches sixty thousand miles, enough to circle the planet 2½ times. Earthly rivers refresh the land with water; the body's stream nourishes and cleanses, delivering food and oxygen to every cell, removing wastes, regulating the human environment. Earth's rivers flow through inorganic rock and sand; the body's river travels through living tissue. The powerful heart that propels this stream and the vessels that guide it are all alive. The human river can regulate its own velocity, its banks widening or narrowing to control the shifting tides. It can change its own course, instantly channeling its swift currents to meet new demands: swimming or sleeping, contemplating, celebrating, running a race or rocking an infant – each alters the flow of this powerful river.

The body's river retains an age-old tie to Earth's waters. Like its prototype the ocean, blood is a crowded sea, teeming with a diverse society of cells that carry out specific tasks and coexist in strict proportions. So critical is this balance that a decline in the population of any one element can endanger life.

The red blood cells constitute about 45% of blood's volume. Every red blood cell contains about 270 million complex proteins to carry oxygen to our body parts. In turn, so many red cells crowd the bloodstream of a single human that stacked, these cells could reach 31,000 miles in the sky.

AMAZING ISN'T IT?

DO YOU KNOW YOUR HEART?

Your heart is the strongest and toughest muscle in your body. In 12 hours, the innate intelligence of your body can generate through your heart enough energy to lift three fully loaded Greyhound Scenicruiser buses one inch off the ground.

Your heart beats usually at about 75 beats per minute... or about 40 million per year. These are only the beats you can feel (your pulse). Actually there are twice that many because your heart is a pump. It pumps blood from your body into your lungs to get renewed oxygen, then pumps it back into your body to supply new food to your tissues. Since both actions happen at the same time you can feel only one beat.

Your heart pumps about 2½ gallons of blood per minute. If you could loan your heart to pump donor blood into pint bottles, it would fill so many bottles in one year that they would stretch from Washington, D.C. to Orlando, Florida.

Your blood is made up of billions of cells floating in a liquid called plasma. It's like a river that flows to every part of your body through your arteries, veins and capillaries.

The red cells in your blood stream are like freight ships that carry oxygen from your lungs to your tissues and take waste gas (carbon dioxide) from your tissues back to your lungs. The white cells in your blood stream are like Coast Guard boats that are always on alert and ready to fight off germs, bacteria and viruses. Other cells called platelets act like dams to shut off the flow of blood whenever you cut yourself. They form tiny threads called fibrin which trap the red cells forming a clot or dam.

A crop of blood only ¹⁄₂₅th of an inch in size contains about 5 million red blood cells, 7,000 white blood cells and thousands of platelets (60,000 of these blood cells could be put on the head of a pin!).

As you can see, your heart is a very active and very important organ of your body. It is under the direct control of the innate intelligence of the body which uses the brain and nerve system to relay messages to and from the heart. For your heart to function at maximum efficiency, it needs a good nerve supply of energy, for without energy from the brain, your heart would just stop beating and you would die. However, sometimes only a small amount of energy is blocked within the nerves and it eventually causes malfunction of the heart leading very often to heart attacks, heart failure, cardiac arrest, hardening of the arteries and high blood pressure.

The Straight Chiropractor, by correcting the blockages to your nerve system, ensures that the right amount of energy will get to your heart and all the parts of your body resulting in a better expression of your innate potential. That is always positive for all the functions of your body, especially your heart!

AMAZING ISN'T IT?

DO YOU KNOW WE HAVE FURNACES WITHIN OUR BODY?

As we each laid in bed this morning, the cells in our bodies burned a minimum amount of oxygen, enough to keep us alive. As we began to stir, our cellular furnaces ignited for the action of the day. When we stood to walk across the room, our bodies doubled their demand. If we exercised, our cells busily consumed 8 to 12 times the oxygen used at night. Some strenuous athletic feats and dire emergencies require such furious energy combustion that our cells burn up to 20 times the oxygen they use at rest.

The heart and blood vessels do more than speed or slow our blood flow to meet these needs. They carry the scarlet stream to different tissues under differing pressures to fuel different actions. Blood rushes to the stomach when we eat, to the lungs and muscles when we swim, to the brain when we read. How does the heart know what to do under these different circumstances? How does it register? How does it respond to needs we do not even consciously recognize ourselves?

Our innate intelligence is the "Wisdom of the Body" which controls all of the above functions and more, using the central nerve system as the tool of communication. As a matter of fact, on constant duty in our brain stems are chemical sensors called carotid bodies that continually "taste" the blood flowing from the heart to tissues, savoring it for the acidic flavor of carbon dioxide and sending the information to our brain to be interpreted. Rising levels of carbon dioxide signal the brain to increase the rate at which our lungs expel it. Other monitors, situated mainly in the aorta and the carotid artery, the major vessel leading to the brain, regulate blood pressure. These stretched receptors activate when a surge of blood, signaling a faster heartbeat, stretches the arteries. The sensors immediately alert the brain, which order the heart rate to slow.

AMAZING ISN'T IT?

DO YOU KNOW YOUR BODY HAS A THERMOSTAT?

Heart rate can rise or fall, but the temperature of the blood must remain constant. A severe drop in body heat can damage cells by inhibiting critical enzyme reactions. Even a mild rise in temperature makes us feverish, and we cannot survive for long if our temperature shoots above 108°F. The innate intelligence of the body monitors its temperature through a thermostat that measures the heat of blood flowing through the brain. If air temperature drops even a fraction of a degree and our blood cools, the autonomic nervous system responds instantly: parasympathetic nerves slow the heart; sympathetic nerves constrict vessels in the skin. Blood flows through deeper pathways, away from the cold air at the skin. When weather turns hot or when we exercise combusting more oxygen and thus generating heat-blood changes course. The sympathetic nerves open arteriole valves, and the blood vessels in our skin act like radiators, cooling the body by casting off heat to the surrounding air.

Continually balancing one another in a state known as homeostasis, an inborn balance in humans controlled by an innate intelligence, the sympathetic and parasympathetic nerves control our blood supply, regulate our pressure, and mediate our temperature. Together, their coordinated actions from the innate intelligence adjust heart rate and blood flow when we stand suddenly, bend over, or even perform acrobatics upside down. If we were to climb from sea level to the thin atmosphere of the Himalayas, the innate intelligence would stimulate the sympathetic nerves which in turn would quicken heart pace to send the oxygen we need to our cells. Breathless and dizzy at first, we would adjust quickly; our bone marrow would step up red cell production, churning out 50% more of the oxygen-carrying cells than at sea level.

Conversely, if we dive underwater, the innate intelligence uses the parasympathetic system to slow the heart, conserving our limited oxygen supply. The sympathetic system constricts blood vessels. This shuts off blood to almost all tissues and changes the cardiovascular system into a shortened circuit that cycles mainly from heart to brain. Arteriole sensors register the rising level of carbon dioxide waste in the blood and flash the brain a signal to surface from the water.

AMAZING ISN'T IT?

DO YOU KNOW YOUR IMMUNE SYSTEM?

Did you know your body had its own "army" ready to defend you against harmful agents such as selective groups of bacteria, virus and germs? This "army" is your immune system, also called your body resistance.

It began to work when you were still within the womb of your mother. The innate intelligence of the body was using the placenta of your mother to manufacture antibodies and interferons that are released within your blood stream to provide you with your first "battalion" to help you fight off potential invaders. Then as you were born and were fed your mother's breast milk (we hope), you received via this human milk your second "battalion" of antibodies. Then three to four weeks later, the innate intelligence of the body began to manufacture its very own "troops" of antibodies and interferons through a small gland called the thymus. Your innate intelligence also manufactures what is called gammaglobulin and immunoglobin (two principal defense agents). Of course your spleen with some other organs and glands are also used by your innate intelligence to produce natural immunity providing you with the most sophisticated warfare weapons against any harmful invaders of your body.

Naturally, for this army to work efficiently, it must be under the command of a great "General": your brain. Your Brain-General sends important orders received from the Chief Commander: your innate intelligence, via a telegraphic system of communication called the nerve system, which is protected within your vertebral column. Sometimes vertebral subluxations interfere with the transmission of the orders sent by your Brain-General creating troubles because your body expresses less of its innate potential. When this occurs, your "army" does not receive the correct orders, it does not perform properly, your resistance decreases and you are prey to invaders (like bacteria, viruses and germs). Sometimes as a result of such a scenario your body becomes sick.

What must you do to regain your health and maintain it? Common sense says that you must repair the interference within the transmission of the orders from your Brain-General.

The Straight Chiropractor corrects vertebral subluxations allowing you to better express your innate potential and providing the battalions and the troops of your "army" (immune system) to once again receive the orders from your Brain-General. Then and only then will your body have a chance to perform properly. And, of course, you will also be fully protected by keeping your resistance high... This is called: prevention.

AMAZING ISN'T IT?

DO YOU KNOW YOUR AUTONOMIC NERVOUS SYSTEM? IS IT SYMPATHETIC OR INVOLUNTARY?

The innate intelligence of your body uses the human brain to preside over every function of your body including those of the heart and blood vessels by designating authority to the autonomic nervous system, two groups that oppose and balance each other. The sympathetic nerves send the heart rate soaring: danger, stress and exertion signal this system to speed the flow of blood. The parasympathetic system counters by slowing the heart down, conserving energy for the demands of everyday life.

The sympathetic nervous system is part of the flight response that primes us for action. You step off a curb; suddenly a speeding taxicab skids around the comer, heading straight for you. The innate intelligence of your body responds to such dangers by signaling the sympathetic nerves to pour out adrenaline and noradrenaline (now called epinephrine and norepinephrine). Both chemicals constrict blood vessels, raise blood pressure, and speed the heart. As the cab bears down, your heart pounds faster and faster, your blood pressure rises, breathing deepens, and muscles tense. You leap for safety and collapse on the sidewalk, sweating and gasping for breath. In extreme emergencies the sympathetic nerves can send the heart rate soaring as high as 200 beats per minute, preparing us for unusual feats of strength or action.

AMAZING ISN'T IT?

IS IT A SYSTEM OF SELF?

Did you know that the immune system is called the system of "self" because it possesses the remarkable ability to tell self from nonself, friend from foe? It recognizes and destroys cancer cells, transplanted tissue cells, and a wide range of organisms, from the minute picornavirus, which are so small that more than a million lined up would fit in the space of an inch to some parasites that are visible to the naked eye. At the same time, it usually respects the body's own tissues, varied as they are. Sometimes the difference between self and foreign is slight, a matter of only a molecule or two, as in the distinction between a normal cell and a cancerous one. How does it know what to respect and what to reject?

Nearly every substance known to mankind bears a chemical identity card made of a characteristic pattern of molecules at its surface. Each of the cells that make up our own tissues and organs carries such an identity card. Because the innate intelligence of the body uses genes to determine the shape and nature of these human selfmakers, they are unique to each individual. Lodged in the outer surface of our cells, they stand as flags of our identity.

The innate intelligence at all times through the immune system surveys the chemical markers of every molecule and cell in the body. Because the marks on our body cells differ from those that brand foreign substances, the immune system can pick out intruders and avoid the reckless execution of friends. If the system recognizes a mark as self, it will usually respect the substance; if it detects a foreign mark, it will launch an attack to destroy the invader.

Any substance that triggers such an attack is called an antigen. Viruses, parasites, fungi, and bacteria can act as antigens. So can blood cells or tissue from another human being and altered self-components, including cancer cells or cells infected by a virus. Even seemingly innocuous substances, such as ragweed pollen, mildew, animal hairs, or house dust, can provoke a full blown attack.

AMAZING ISN'T IT?

WHY DO WE HAVE LYMPH NODES?

Most of us have felt the glands in our necks enlarge and grow tender when we have the flu, or those under the arm or near the elbow swell when a finger becomes infected. These glands are actually lymph nodes.

Usually one or more of these nodes lie in the pathway of the lymphatic vessels and filter the lymph on its way to the bloodstream. In each node, a labyrinth of channels weaves through a dense webbing of tissue divided into compartments. Each compartment houses a distinct population of white blood cells. As the incoming lymph trickles through the channels of the node, some particles get caught in the webbing or fall prey to white blood cells. In this way, the nodes filter out foreign chemicals, particles and microorganisms before they enter the bloodstream. This function was discovered during an autopsy performed on a heavily tattooed sailor. His lymph nodes showed traces of ink.

When an un-welcomed organism arrives at a node from a site of infection, the innate intelligence commands the brain to send chemoelectrical impulses down the spinal cord, in through the nerves to stimulate the node which swells as the white blood cells within divide and multiply in response to the invader.

AMAZING ISN'T IT?

LET'S ILLUMINATE THE IMMUNE SYSTEM... SHALL WE?

Unlike the digestive or circulatory systems, the immune system is not contained within a set of organs or network of vessels: Its elements permeate nearly every part of the body.

Imagine the components of this immune system glowing from within. Its key operators, a class of white blood cells known as lymphocytes, appear from head to toe. Like minute, twinkling lights, a trillion or more lymphocytes illuminate the blood, lungs, liver, stomach, and nearly every other body tissue. So do scavenging white blood cells called phagocytes (from greek, phagein: to eat).

Against the dark silhouette of a human form, two of the systems organs glow bright: the thymus, a small, two lobed organ just behind the breastbone, and the soft, gelatinous tissue of the marrow deep within our long bones. In these primary lymphoid organs, lymphocytes grow and develop.

Also glowing are the secondary lymphoid organs, the sites where lymphocytes are stored and where some immune responses take place. These include the spleen, an organ in the upper abdomen that filters blood, and the lymph nodes, pulpy clumps of tissue, as well as the tonsils, adenoids, appendix, and the Peyer's patches, bits of lymphoid tissue embedded in the walls of the small intestine.

A network of lymphatic vessels connects these widely dispersed organs. The vessels carry lymph, a colorless fluid that leaks from the bloodstream, collects between our cells, and then seeps into the small lymphatic capillaries, whose walls allow fluid in but prevent it from escaping again. Lymph, like blood, transports the cells of the immune system, as well as foreign substances that find their way into body tissues.

The network of vessels begin in a multitude of thin walled capillaries that branch throughout the tissues. Like small tributaries that feed into major waterways, these tiny tubes drain into larger and larger vessels. From the top of the scalp, they run down through the neck; from the hands and feet, they flow up through the limbs to the torso. In the lower part of the neck, the biggest vessels pour their contents into two large lymphatic channels. These channels, in turn, ultimately converge with veins that lead into the heart.

Unlike the blood circulatory system, the lymphatic system has no pump to keep its vital fluid in continual motion. Instead, body movements and muscle contractions squeeze the vessels, propelling lymph along its course.

AMAZING ISN'T IT?

IS THAT A BIG EATER?

The macrophage sometimes originates in the bone marrow. Known as monocytes in their immature form, these cells leave the marrow, travel through the bloodstream for a few days, and then migrate into the tissues.

There they mature into macrophages, or "big eaters", professional scavengers with a nearly insatiable appetite for undesirable cells. Many macrophages settle at the common site of entry for undesired microorganisms, including the tissues of the lungs, digestive system and circulatory system. When a macrophage receives a warning signal from infected cells or tissues, the innate intelligence commands that macrophage to develop still further, acquiring even more sophisticated cellular machinery.

Unlike neutrophils, which live for only a few days, mature macrophages live in the body's tissues for months, perhaps even years. Some act as janitors, sweeping up dirt, damaged tissue, and aged cells. Each day, the macrophages in a single human body consume more than 300 billion dead or dying red blood cells. In the lungs, macrophages continuously clean the surfaces of the air sacs, mopping up the bits and pieces of matter that find their way past the nostril hairs and cilia of the respiratory tract. They can even clear lung tissues darkened by tar from tobacco smoke. As long as they do not have to cope with additional smoke pollution, macrophages can eventually restore the lung's normal appearance. Therefore, it is never too late to quit smoking.

AMAZING ISN'T IT?

HOW MUCH DO WE KNOW?

Many of you right now must be wondering how amazing your body truly is. You have much reason to wonder, because the information that is presented to you within this book is only a very small fraction of the totality of function of the human body. According to Professor Leandre Poisson, who was the director of the Academie Francaise of Science, scientists know about $\frac{1}{1000}$th of 1% of the human body. Therefore, much is involved and yet, we as human beings manage to live rather well. It is due to the innate intelligence in each of us that we can go through life with relative ease.

When you come in for a spinal check, you help your body to communicate within itself in an orderly manner. Adjustments correct interferences to your nerve system which is located within your spinal column. The chemo-electrical impulses travel down your spine and out your nerves to activate your entire body. When these impulses are free from interferences, your body's ability to function properly increases tremendously, thus allowing you to enjoy wellness throughout.

The past few pages have been dealing with the immune system of the body. What a remarkable organization your immune system is! Macrophages for example, use some of the enzymes they produce to cut their way through the thick tangle of fibers, proteins, and debris at the site of infection as they move toward the microbes. Unlike the neutrophils, which can consume only one big meal, activated macrophages engulf numerous intruders, digest them, and move on with relentless energy to pursue more prey, sometimes destroying up to a hundred bacteria before they expire. As the struggle continues, dead tissue, digested microorganisms, spent phagocytes, and debris may ooze from the wound as pus.

AMAZING ISN'T IT?

ORGANISMS THAT EAT CELLS?

Patrolling phagocytes, the body's "eating cells", often intercept foreign substances that find their way into the body's lymph, blood, or tissues. The two most common types of phagocytes, the smaller, short-lived neutrophils, and the larger, tougher macrophages, seek out viruses, bacteria, fungi, protozoa, and other invaders. Doesn't this make you feel good to know that this kind of wonderful system is working within you right now?

Each day, some 100 billion neutrophils leave the bone marrow and enter the bloodstream. Nearly half of them circulate with the blood; the rest, known as the marginal pool, cling to the walls of the blood vessels. Almost any kind of stress to tissues in the body triggers a rise in the number of blood-borne neutrophils. During severe infection, their number may increase more than fivefold, some originating from the marginal pool, others arising fresh from the bone marrow. At the appropriate signal from the innate intelligence, the neutrophils leave the bloodstream and migrate into the tissues to pursue invading microorganisms.

AMAZING ISN'T IT?

IS THERE WAR?

Within minutes of infection, the innate intelligence summons a wave of neutrophils which arrives at the site, the advance guard of the body's professional "eating cells". Each neutrophil convulsed by the chemical signals sent by the innate intelligence, thrusts a portion of its cell body between the crevices in the blood vessel walls, squeezes through, and slithers toward the microbes. A struggles ensues.

The bacteria, dodging their attackers, spew powerful toxins that can disable or kill the neutrophils and surrounding cells. A persistent neutrophil seizes a bacterium and wraps a portion of its own cell membrane around the microbe. By sucking the membrane inward, deep into its body, the neutrophil creates a miniature sac for its prey. Once imprisoned within the white blood cell, the bacterium may writhe and twist and disgorge its poisons in a last-ditch effort to escape its captor. But now the neutrophil dispatches its own weapons, small bags, each filled with a load of digestive juices and microbe-killing agents, which release their contents on the bacterium. The powerful juices quickly digest the prey. Each neutrophil may engulf and destroy up to 25 bacteria, but its efforts take a heavy toll. At the end of its bout, the neutrophil dies from the accumulation of its own digestive juices and the poisons released by the bacteria.

Neutrophils last for only a short time, but the innate intelligence of the body sends in a steady stream of reinforcement. More neutrophils arrive to join the struggle.

AMAZING ISN'T IT?

ARE THEY BODY GUARDS?

Within the amazing body, the innate intelligence will make sure that its organism is very well protected. Everything we encounter bears a rich load of foreign material. The air we breathe carries dirt, exhaust fumes, and bits of debris, including pollen grains from hundreds of different plants.

Dust that settles on the furniture and floors of our homes often holds human or pet dander (tiny scales that flake from hair, skin or feathers) as well as microscopic cousins of the spider called mites. Even the food we eat harbors bacteria, mold and fungal spores. Fortunately, the immune system does not have to confront the bulk of these substances. A set of first-line defenses keeps most foreign material outside the body, away from its inner tissues. These defenses include the body's tough outer covering of skin and membranes; its protective reflexes, such as coughing and sneezing; and a variety of fluids that wash over its surfaces.

As long as the skin remains uninjured, it holds the body's insides in and keeps the rest of the world safely out. This remarkable organ also has the ability to regenerate. Despite daily scratching, ripping, tanning, burning and exposure to irritating soaps and drying heat, skin retains its integrity. The innate intelligence, through many organs and glands, constantly relubricates and replenishes its outer surface, the epidermis, and heals ruptures in its deeper layer, the dermis.

AMAZING ISN'T IT?

ARE THEY TRAPPERS? GARBAGE COLLECTORS?

Though we rarely think of them as such, the membranes that line the body's internal surfaces, including the respiratory and digestive tracts, are as much a part of the body's protective covering as the skin is. These membranes encounter microbes and other foreign material in quantity, and therefore, must be armed with a set of defenses equal to the skin's.

In the respiratory tract, (the air passages that lead to the lungs, such as the nose, trachea, and bronchial tubes) a collection of highly efficient mechanisms work around-the-clock to ensure that only moist, temperate air, almost free of debris, reaches the lungs' air sacs. During the course of a day in a city, we inhale up to 17,000 pints of air. That air contains some 20 billion particles of foreign material, including dirt, dust and chemicals, most of which never make it to the lungs.

Airborne matter that enters the nose must pass through a trap of stiff nostril hairs that catches many of the larger particles. Just past this trap, the direction of the airstream shifts abruptly with the curve of the bones in the nasal passage, forcing some of the larger particles to collide with the wall of the pharynx. Here, the innate intelligence uses tonsils and adenoids, (strategically placed tissues containing agents of the immune system) to trap foreign material and see to its destruction.

AMAZING ISN'T IT?

CAN WE TALK ABOUT A VIRUS?

Let us take a look at an invasion of the body by a cold virus. Consider the cooperative efforts of the body's immune cells and molecules in an encounter with a rhinovirus, the agent that is involved in 30% of all colds. Like other viruses, the rhinovirus consists of a strand of genetic material encased in a protein coat. It enters the body through the mucus membranes in our nose, throat and eyes. Latching on to the surface of its host cell, the viral agent penetrates the membrane of its target and injects its own genetic material into the cell body.

Once inside the host, this minute fraction of genetic information swiftly tries to divert the cell's machinery to the production of new virus particles, or virions. However, as long as the resistance of the body is kept high, this diversion is not successful and nothing happens to the body. If the central nerve system is interfered with by a spinal subluxation, as many as a thousand new virions may come bursting out of the now dead and wasted body cell, ready to attack healthy cells. In most cases, the body responds immediately to the destruction of that first infected cell.

Before the body's beleaguered cells succumb to their viral attackers, they release a substance called interferon. This powerful chemical is used by the innate intelligence of the body to alert nearby cells to the presence of the virus. These neighboring cells then produce a protein that prevents the viruses from multiplying within them, thus limiting the spread of the infection.

AMAZING ISN'T IT?

WHAT IS HOMEOSTASIS?

The body's internal and external surfaces support communities of microscopic allies. Populations of resident flora, or friendly bacteria, live on the skin, in the mouth, stomach, and lower intestines. They also inhabit the ears and other parts of the body. The innate intelligence of the body controls and coordinates every function of your body including the presence of these microorganisms and in doing so, prevents virulent (dangerous) organisms from multiplying.

Any dangerous microbe trying to settle on the skin must contend with a well-entrenched colony of bacteria, with nearly 20 million microorganisms per square inch, some of which make life unpleasant for newcomers. Certain friendly bacteria produce fatty acids that hinder the growth of other strains of bacteria and several kinds of fungi. The bacteria Escherichia coli, which live in the intestinal tract and work as part of our nutritional system, simply use up the nutrients that other, less favorable types of bacteria require to live and produce, therefore starving out their competition.

Experience with antibiotics has demonstrated the dangers of disturbing the microbial life that normally inhabits the body. Long-term use of these substances can wipe out friendly and neutral germs as well as hostile ones... with disastrous results. Once rid of their competitors, dangerous microbes quickly establish themselves sometimes forcing the innate intelligence of the body to produce certain chemicals in order to re-establish a certain balance called homeostasis. However, during this healing period, the body may experience strange and unusual symptoms (such as diarrhea, vomiting, etc.) which are good but oftentimes cause unnecessary worries on the part of the individual.

The body's physical barriers and other first line defenses most often prevent microbes and other foreign matter from entering the body's inner tissues... but not always. Bacteria sometimes enter the deeper layers of the skin through a cut in the finger. Viruses slip through the lining of the respiratory and digestive tracts, penetrating the lungs or intestines. Such invading microorganisms usually encounter the full force of the immune system and are destroyed on the spot.

AMAZING ISN'T IT?

DO YOU KNOW THE INFLAMMATION RESPONSE?

A splinter breaking the skins sets off a battle within the body – the inflammatory response which is under the direct control of the innate intelligence of the body.

Innate intelligence sends mast cells at the site of the injury to release chemicals that affect nearby capillaries. Then it commands the tiny blood vessels to expand their walls and become more porous. As additional blood flows into the area, the skin reddens and heats up. Blood serum seeping from the leaky capillaries makes the wounded tissue swell and grow tender.

Within an hour, the innate intelligence sends white blood cells, called neutrophils, to mobilize and to fight invading microbes that rode in on the splinter. These small cells speed to the battle site, slither through capillary walls, and gobble up bacteria.

Later, larger white blood cells, the macrophages, begin to arrive. These scavengers sweep over the site, wrapping their finger-like pseudopods around the bacteria and eating them. Macrophages also devour dead neutrophils and other debris.

For hours, often days, the white blood cells muster forces to defeat the invading horde and prepare the way for the process of healing and repair.

Can you sense the healing process within your body? That is exactly how it works.

AMAZING ISN'T IT?

ARE THEY ANTI-BODIES OR PRO-BODY?

The innate intelligence coordinates the functions of the human body, including the manufacturing of millions of antibodies. All antibodies are divided into classes according to their structure and the defensive tasks they perform. One group fights bacteria with great efficiency. These antibodies, because of their large size, are restricted to working almost entirely within the blood vessels. The members of another group, built in a way that allows them to cross the placenta, provide the fetus and newborn baby with protection until the body's own immune system becomes fully developed.

In most cases, the various parts of the immune system: T-cells, B-cells, and phagocytes work together under the control of the innate intelligence of the body. B-cells make up one class of lymphocytes. The second class, known as T-cells, mature in the thymus gland (T stands for thymus). Some are "killer" cells and they kill invading agents. Other T-cells regulate the strength of the immune response. Those known as "helper" cells secrete substances that turn on antibody production and stimulate the immune system in times of need; those known as "suppressor" cells produce chemicals that turn off antibody production and suppress the action to other T-cells. These regulator cells ensure an appropriate response to any single invader.

In people with the condition knows as AIDS (acquired immunodeficiency syndrome), the normal ratio of helper to suppressor T-cells is disturbed. The AIDS virus attacks helper T-cells, preventing them from carrying out one of their regular duties to activate the immune system when a threat arises. This breakdown in normal communication between immune cells leaves the body virtually undefended, that those who are infected from AIDS become victims of a rare skin cancer called Kaposi's sarcoma, life-threatening pneumonia, and other various serious infections.

No single organ or set of organs orchestrates their defensive operations. However, the central nerve system (this is the system that the adjustments allow to work without interference) is used by the innate intelligence to provide the mental impulses necessary for proper communications amongst the cells of the immune system which "talk" to each other in a language of chemical signals, a language with a large vocabulary and a complex grammar. Each cell sends and receives several different messages which are under the supervision of the innate intelligence. Each message, well timed and precisely directed, stimulates or inhibits other cells or regulates their activities. As the innate intelligence of the body molds its defense against a particular invader, the pattern of signals shifts slightly to suit moment-to-moment needs. The result is a delicately balanced, sensitive system of defense powerful enough to destroy or neutralize the effects of nearly any foreign intruder.

AMAZING ISN'T IT?

ARE T-CELLS AND B-CELLS DESTROYERS?

Within your body, there exist T-cells with receptors designed to recognize all kinds of viruses and when the innate intelligence of the body has determined which kind of particular virus is at work, the T-cells respond by multiplying. Newly formed T-cells secrete a chemical that attracts more macrophages to the site of infection and holds them there.

Some T-cells travel through the bloodstream to nearby lymph nodes to spread the word of the invasion. There they contact B-cells and killer T-cells genetically programmed to react to any particular virus.

The killer T-cells leave the node and migrate to the site of infection. Using their specialized receptors, they attach to the surface of the infected cells and this happens under direct control of the innate intelligence of the body. Less than a minute after contact, the T-cell delivers a chemical signal to the target cell, which results in its destruction hours later. Meanwhile the T-cell moves on to destroy other infected cells.

AMAZING ISN'T IT?

DO WE HAVE GATE KEEPERS?

Continuing our study of the immune system, we now realize that unlike phagocytes, lymphocytes have the ability to recognize the precise identity of virtually any antigen, or foreign substance, millions of different molecules.

The innate intelligence can tell with the use of lymphocytes an infected liver cell from its healthy counterpart or a cancerous body cell from a normal one by recognizing small differences in the cells' chemical markers. Differences between influenza virus and a smallpox virus or a staphyloccus bacterium and an Escherichia coli can be noticed by specific recognition sites called receptors that each lymphocyte carries on its surface.

Although the above mentioned terms are complex, let us remember that the innate intelligence is incredibly capable of keeping our bodies functioning properly as long as it has a good nerve supply, proper nutrition, regular exercise and a positive mental attitude.

AMAZING ISN'T IT?

WHAT ABOUT THE ASSISTANCE OF FEVER?

When confronted by some organisms, macrophages produce a substance called interleukin-1, which triggers fever. Once released by the macrophage, the interleukin-1 travels through the bloodstream to the tiny portion of the brain that controls body temperature a small cluster of neurons deep within the hypothalamus.

The innate intelligence through this chemical prompts the temperature regulator to set a new body temperature. Nerve impulses from the hypothalamus then spark the body's heat conserving mechanisms, blood vessels in the skin constrict, preventing heat loss; muscles contract, causing shivering. We cover up with sweaters and blankets until the body temperature reaches its new set point. As long as the fever remains mild (up to 106°F) and does not persist for more than a few days (up to 10 days), the raised temperature appears to increase the efficiency of the body's infection-fighting agent. The antiviral substance interferon operates more effectively. Phagocytes attack their prey with more speed and vigor. Fever may even increase production of T-cells which you now know are responsible for the immune response within the body.

As the lymphocytes, phagocytes, and antibodies begin to overcome the virus, the innate intelligence uses suppressor T-cells to signal the defenders to bring their efforts to a halt. Your head clears, your runny nose dries up, you can swallow easily again. All of that without the help of medications.

AMAZING ISN'T IT?

WHAT ARE GENETIC MARKERS?

The cells and chemicals of the immune system work together to protect the body from outside threats. The innate intelligence controls all systems of the body. How does the immune system handle threats that arise from within?

Every day an adult produces some 300 billion new cells. They usually divide as they should, but sometimes, vertebral subluxations can sabotage the communications between the brain and tissues to an extent that can rearrange the genes that regulate normal cell growth and differentiation. When this occurs, that single cell may begin to divide uncontrollably, multiplying and joining to form a colony of mutant cells, a malignant tumor.

When a body cell becomes cancerous, its membrane may change slightly, so that it bears markers somewhat different from the body's own. Ordinarily, agents of the immune system will recognize and react to the new markers, eliminating the mutant cell.

I believe that the cellular part of the immune system has developed originally as a surveillance mechanism for cancer cells. In the course of our life, our bodies develop a slightly refined system for recognizing subtle distinctions between self and nonself.

That is why the rejection of a transplant is the price we pay for possessing such an efficient system of surveillance. If a surgeon transplants a patch of skin from one part of a patient's body to another part, the graft is usually accepted as self. But if the surgeon attempts to transplant skin from brother to sister, the borrowed tissue grows puffy, inflamed, and irritated. Eventually it drops off. Even though the donor and recipient are blood related, the graft is rejected as foreign by the innate intelligence's immune system of the body.

AMAZING ISN'T IT?

CAN WE HAVE AN INTIMATE CONVERSATION?

The immune system works remarkably well for most of us most of the time. Just how it works differs from person to person. However, we know that the immune system is controlled by the innate intelligence of the body and that it reflects the life history and individuality of its owner. How any one person will meet a given challenge depends on many things, especially the integrity of the nerve system and its freedom from subluxation.

In general, the immune system is subject to the perpetual cycles of change within the body. It is a system of balance, of dynamic equilibrium, intimately connected to the nerve system. Evidence suggests that immune cells themselves send messages to the brain. Nerve cells and immune cells seem to engage in two-way conversations. Some immune cells have receptors on their membranes for neuropeptides which are chemicals produced by the brain. That is why it is good to have a spinal column well adjusted at all times.

For the most part, these systems work with the body's other cells and tissues, maintaining stability and balance within, preserving our most precious possession: health.

AMAZING ISN'T IT?

DO YOU KNOW YOUR SKIN?

The skin is the body's largest and one of its most complex organs. Spread flat, it would cover approximately 18 square feet, every square inch of which includes about 3 feet of blood vessels, 12 feet of nerves, 100 sweat glands and more than 3 million cells. Without this natural spacesuit we would be prey to all sorts of deadly bacteria and, in any case, would quickly perish from loss of body heat.

There are two basic parts to your skin. The surface called the epidermis which is the part that gets rubbed off when you skin a knuckle or a knee. The next layer below called the dermis is where most of the blood vessels reside. In order to bleed, a cut must be deep enough to reach the dermis.

Also there are two kinds of glands in your skin. Sweat glands, (about 2 millon) through which you perspire in order to get rid of liquid waste matter and to cool you off as the sweat evaporates on the skin. Oil glands waterproof your skin, preventing it from becoming too dry. They also keep your hair smooth and glossy.

All of the functions of the skin are directly controlled by the innate intelligence of the body which uses the brain and the nerve system to coordinate them. Since the skin has such an important role, it is imperative that the nerve system be free from vertebral subluxations at all times, because they interfere with the flow of mental impulses, thus allowing the skin and other parts of the body to mal-function and develop symptoms (like rashes, redness, dryness) and diseases such as eczema, psoriasis, dandruff, acne and skin cancer.

By correcting vertebral subluxations, the Straight Chiropractor allows a better expression of the innate potential of the body, thereby insuring a good nerve supply to the skin and all other parts of the body.

AMAZING ISN'T IT?

DO YOU KNOW MORE ABOUT YOUR SKIN?

The skin always fascinates me in so many ways. Did you know that beneath a "forest of hair" the terrain of skin throbs with life? One square inch may hold 650 sweat glands, 20 blood vessels, and more than 1,000 nerve endings.

On the top layer, or epidermis, a sheet of dead cells forms a horny shield of keratin. Many microorganisms perish on contact with this surface, which is bathed in salty sweat and acidic, oily sebum. Other microbial invaders fall away as surface cells dry up and flake off. The shed skin is replenished by a living layer of basal cells that divide and move to the surface.

The innate intelligence of the body will use sebaceous glands to pump out the sebum that lubricates skin and hair. To limit the damaging effects of sun, melanocytes inject surface cells with the pigment melanin. This is why we must be prudent while sunbathing and use our knowledge and be sensible. While the natural sunlight is absolutely necessary for proper synthesis of vitamin D through natural ultra-violet rays from the sun, the artificial use of these rays can be very harmful.

Deeper down, the thick mass of connective tissue called the dermis, and lower lying fat cells, act as shock absorbers, padding the body's inner tissues from outside blows.

The innate intelligence of the body uses blood vessels to help regulate temperature, widening or constricting them, to release or conserve heat. On cold days the erector pili muscle contracts, causing the hair to stand up. In animals their reaction traps an insulating layer of warm air near the skin. In humans it results only in goose bumps.

Snaking through this environment is a warning system of nerve fibers that terminate in endings, either free or enclosed in corpuscles. This network tingles in response to touch, pressure, heat and cold, alerting the brain to the world outside.

AMAZING ISN'T IT?

IS IT HEAT OR COLD?

The senses of touch, pressure, heat, cold and pain are called the cutaneous senses, from cutis, the Latin word for "skin". The tongue has a high density of these receptors and a high degree of sensitivity. The center of the back is more sparsely endowed with receptors, and shows a correspondingly lower response. A blind person reads Braille with the fingertips, not the knuckles or the heal of the hand. There are some 640,000 cutaneous senses receptors distributed over the body's surface.

Everywhere in the skin (and in some other tissues) is one kind of receptor fibers known as free nerve endings. These have no specialized structure enclosing them. They react to touch and pressure more slowly than other receptors. Another type, Meissner's corpuscles, are nerve endings where the fibers are compartmentalized in capsules. These exist abundantly in the ridges of the fingertips (9,000 to the square inch), in the lips, the tongue tip, the palm, the sole of the foot, and the genital organs. They respond and adapt quickly, within milliseconds, to even a light brush. Merkel's disks carry continuing signals such as sustained pressure. They lie along the edges of the tongue and in some hairy parts of the body. The hair end organ responses to the slightest movement of a hair, even before anything touches the skin, by means of nerve fibers that entwine the base of the hair. Ruffini's end organs, deep below the skin surface, contain many branched fibers, encapsulated nerve endings that respond steadily to heavy, continuous pressure. Other encapsulated receptors, Pacinian corpuscles, lie in the tissue near joints, in the mammary glands, in the genitals, and in some deep tissues like the intestinal walls. Because of their onion-like layers of connective tissue, they react to vibrations and pressure changes within a fraction of a second. Finding the receptors for cold and warmth has not been easy. Once, good candidates were the Krause end bulb and the Ruddine end organ but no longer. Cold receptors, examined under microscope, look just like free nerve endings.

AMAZING ISN'T IT?

HOW DO WE GET BIGGER AND BIGGER?

Have you ever asked yourself: "How do I grow and develop?" Nursery rhymes talk of sugar and spice and all things nice, but little girls, just like puppy dog tails and little boys for that matter, are made of cells. The human body of an adult consists of about 70,000 trillion cells, all derived from just one cell, the fertilized egg.

Growth involves either an increase in size of existing cells or the creation of new ones by cell division. Both processes are at work throughout life, but one tends to dominate at any given stage of development.

Growth is not a simple story of cells getting bigger and bigger. They cannot. There is a physical limit to their size. Many cells are ball shaped. As a cell enlarges, its volume increases at a rate greater than its surface area. Since all materials needed for the cell to carry out its activity must cross the surface membrane, the surface area of the cell will ultimately limit how much it can absorb. Some cells overcome this size restriction either by altering their shape to an elongated form, like a nerve cell, or to a flattened shape, like a skin cell or by using hair-like projections to increase absorption the way an intestinal cell does. These adaptations enable a cell to increase its surface area without increasing its volume.

AMAZING ISN'T IT?

ARE THERE REALLY GROWTH SPURTS?

Some parts of the body grow faster than others, which explains why a baby's proportions are very different from those of an adult. A newborn's head accounts for one-quarter of its body length; the brain is relatively large and well developed. By contrast, the head of an adult is less than one-seventh of total body length. A baby's legs are about one-third its length, while an adult's legs are half the body's length.

We do not grow at a constant rate. The most rapid rate occurs before birth, when in the space of nine months, the fetus increases in weight about 2.4 billion times. After birth, two spurts of growth, one in the first two years and again at puberty, are separated by a slower, more steady rate, where height increases by two to three inches a year and weight increases by five to six pounds. By their first birthdays, babies usually weigh three times their birth weight and have grown in height by 50 percent. Adolescents may grow four to six inches a year.

We must note that growth is very much under the direct control of the innate intelligence of the body.

AMAZING ISN'T IT?

DO YOU KNOW YOUR LOCOMOTOR SYSTEM?
FUSION OF BONES OR BONES' FUSION?

Until adulthood the long bones, elongated bones in the fingers, arms, legs and hips grow quickly by expanding at each end. These growth centers contain gristle-like cartilage cells that create layer upon layer of new bone tissue. Once the cartilage cells stop dividing, the growth centers harden into bone, marking the end of growth in that region. Most growth centers, such as those in the femur and tibia of the leg, have ossified by the age of 17 to 20 years. The breastbone is one of the last bones to stop growing, around age 25.

By the time you grow from infancy to adulthood, you will have about 144 fewer bones: The innate intelligence of the body sees to it that the 350 or so bones in a newborn gradually fuse into the approximately 206 bones in the adult skeleton. The number of bones varies because some people have an extra pair of ribs or fewer vertebrae in the spine, etc.

Why do we stop growing when we have reached less than a third of our life expectancy? Aquatic species such as mollusks, crustaceans, and some fish grow indefinitely. One giant clam weighed 600 pounds and may have been 100 years old; giant squid can grow to 50 feet; a giant 2,800 pound turtle has been reported. The major reason for growth is that the water helps support the weight. But land-dwelling creatures have to support their bony weight themselves, so their innate intelligence has evolved ways of limiting their size.

AMAZING ISN'T IT?

DO YOU KNOW YOUR HORMONAL SYSTEM?
IS IT A DOMINO EFFECT?

The innate intelligence of the body coordinates the endocrine functions and allows the secretion of hormones to control how fast we grow. Scattered through the body like tiny islands, the endocrine glands affect every aspect of our growth, physical and mental development, reproduction, and cell repair. Endocrine glands act on organs or certain types of tissues located in other parts of the body by releasing hormones, or chemical regulators, into the bloodstream. These hormones come in contact with every cell, but only certain ones called target cells, will respond to any given hormone. Once the hormone molecules bind to receptor-proteins in the target cells the hormones set off a cascade or reactions, causing specific chemical reactions to speed up or slow down.

Two different mechanisms relay the information brought by the hormone to the target cell. Some hormones enter the cell and bind to a receptor-protein in the cytoplasm, the gelatin-like substance encasing the nucleus. Together, the hormone and receptor move to the nucleus, bind to the chromosome, and cause the cell to synthesize certain proteins. Other hormones do not enter the cell at all. They bind to receptor-proteins on the cell's surface and trigger the release of a second messenger in the cytoplasm. It is this compound that then initiates the cell's response to the hormones.

AMAZING ISN'T IT?

DO HORMONES HAVE AN INNER ROOM?

Before puberty begins, hormones play a major part in regulating growth. The growth hormone, somatotropin, is used as the main substance by the innate intelligence of the body to control height. It is one of several hormones secreted by the pituitary gland which dangles from the base of the brain, just above the roof of the mouth. Somatotropin stimulates bone and muscle growth, maintains the normal rate of protein synthesis in all body cells, and speeds the release of fats as an energy source for growth. The pituitary also releases thyroid-stimulating hormone whenever the innate intelligence commands it. This chemical causes the thyroid gland, set like a pinkish bow tie on the windpipe, to secrete hormones that influence general metabolism, especially the growth of the brain, bones and teeth.

It is tempting to refer to the pituitary as the master gland because it is used to regulate the release of hormones from other glands. But the pituitary is actually controlled by a region in the middle underside of the brain known as the hypothalamus (Greek for "under the inner room"). A special set of blood vessels connects these two glands and carries messages from one to the other. The innate intelligence of the body uses the hypothalamus to release chemicals which tumble half an inch to the pituitary and tell it to secrete its hormones. When hormones from other glands reach high levels in the bloodstream, they send a message to the hypothalamus to stop releasing chemicals. This in turn slows the release of hormones from the pituitary.

AMAZING ISN'T IT?

CENTRAL NERVOUS SYSTEM:
WHAT KIND OF TRANSMISSION?

Transmission (trans mish' en) 1. A sending over; passing on; passing along; letting through. 2. Something transmitted. 3a. Part of an automobile that transmits power from the engine to the rear axle or sometimes the front axle. 3b. Sets of gears that determine the relative speed. 4. Passage through space of electromagnetic waves from a transmitting station to a receiving station or stations. (The World Book Dictionary Encyclopedia, Volume 2, 1964, p.2072).

The brain sends impulses, conveys messages, passes on a created force to all the organs, cells, and tissues of the body. In essence, the brain is the innate intelligence center that governs the state and the actions of each individual body cell. Sounds great, right? However, there can be a problem; there may be interference with the transmission of impulses through the body's transportation system (the nerve passages, of course). This interference with transmission results in dysfunction or dis-ease (lack of ease).

Put yourself in first gear; understand that your brain is the center of the body's operations, thus the name "Central Nervous System" as we know it. Your brain is the boss. It was the first organ to appear after conception. It controlled every aspect of the development of your body, and to this day commands every function, even those that you don't know about! The body has (thanks to the brain) the capacity to fight infection and treat and cure disease. What a wonderful invention! Who can beat it? Do you even want to try?

AMAZING ISN'T IT?

WHAT ARE EFFERENT TRANSMISSIONS?

Efferent means "from brain cell to tissue cell", therefore we expect that efferent transmission is the passing on of chemoelectrical impulses from the brain cells to the tissue cells of the body.

As the center of the innate intelligence, the brain creates a mental image, transforms it to energy, and distributes it via the nervous system to specific tissue cells. The brain, with its ability to create energy, enables the tissue cells receiving the impulse to be intelligent. Thus, we have expression, function, or coordinated movement as a result of efferent transmission.

So this is the unison of intelligence and matter, matter meaning any tissue cell or group of cells. Without intelligence, matter cannot be functional. In other words, without efferent transmission, life will cease to exist. The creative ability of the innate intelligence has no limitations, however, our limited perception does indeed put boundaries on our capacity to think.

AMAZING ISN'T IT?

WHAT ARE AFFERENT TRANSMISSIONS?

Afferent means "from tissue cell to brain cell" and therefore afferent transmission is the sending of impulses from the tissue cells at the periphery (or outer region) of the body to the brain cells at the center.

Thus, every tissue cell maintains a communication with the brain by the process of afferent transmission. This receiving and collecting of information by the brain enables the brain cells to perform such functions as sensation, interpretation and impression. Afferent transmission is the means by which the brain interprets sight, smell, touch, pain, etc.

At the meeting of the transmitted energy with the brain cells, the innate intelligence changes the energy to mental power. Without afferent transmission, the brain does not know what occurred in the tissue cells. Therefore, without afferent transmission, there is no sensation. There is no sight. There is no feeling. There is no means by which the brain can monitor the response of the organs and tissues of the body.

AMAZING ISN'T IT?

AFFERENT & EFFERENT TRANSMISSIONS: WHY SO IMPORTANT?

Imagine that you have just finished running a tub of hot water for a relaxing bath. Now you are ready to hop in. You know that you want to lift your leg into the tub, and so your brain creates a mental image and transforms it into energy, sending a message to the tissue cells in order to lift your leg, giving life and mobility so that you are able to raise and lower your leg. The result is a coordinated movement.

Back to your bath. You've just placed your foot into the tub, but uh-oh, the water is scalding. The afferent nerves are sending impulses to the brain telling it that the water is too hot. Even before you have the chance to say "OUCH!", your brain has created another mental image, transformed it into energy, and sent a message by way of efferent nerves, once again allowing your foot to be pulled rapidly out of the hot water.

Without efferent transmission, you would not have been able to lift your leg in the first place. And without afferent transmission, your brain would not have received messages that the water was too hot, and therefore would not have sent messages to remove it from the water. The result would have been burned skin.

AMAZING ISN'T IT?

ARE THE TRANSMISSIONS ROADBLOCKS?

Recently we have talked about transmissions, what it means, what it does, and how it affects our bodies. The brain is the tool used by the innate intelligence within our bodies. By way of efferent nerves, the brain gives life to the body. And by way of afferent nerves, the brain maintains communication to those cells to which it has given life, monitoring them, so to speak.

So all is well, right? WRONG! The spinal column is the bone structure that protects the spinal cord. Between each segment, nerves branch from the spinal cord to send electrical impulses to all of the tissues and organs in the body. However, if one or more of these segments is displaced, pressure is placed on a nerve and therefore there is interference with the transmission of electrical impulses within the body. This means that the innate intelligence has reached a roadblock, and cannot send life to all of the organs and tissues in the body. This condition is called a subluxation. Unfortunately, our bodies are very susceptible to subluxations. They are caused by any type of stress: physical, chemical, emotional, and can lead to any type of disease or disorder. For instance: a fall, whiplash sustained in an automobile accident, chemicals from over-the-counter or prescription medications, alcohol, high pressure careers, little falls you took as a child, and even being born can cause subluxations that can lead to serious illnesses later on in life.

So, what do you do to eliminate or decrease the possibility of illness due to interference of the spinal nerves? That's easy... have your spine checked periodically by a Straight Chiropractor!

AMAZING ISN'T IT?

CAN YOU SHOW ME A SUBLUXATION?

As stated previously, cycles are the basis for our very existence. The interference with the cycle can cause disorder, dysfunction, disease and death. The single interfering factor within our body that can lead to serious consequences all the time is a subluxation.

A subluxation by definition is the movement of a spinal bone (called a vertebra) out of its proper position, so that it puts pressure on a nerve, thus interfering with the normal flow of impulses through the spine to and from all the organs and tissues of the body.

The moment a subluxation occurs, it decreases the ability of an organ to function to its fullest potential. The organ that is affected depends on the nerve that is "pinched". For instance, if a nerve leading to the stomach is pinched, the stomach, not receiving the proper signals from the brain, may overproduce some digestive acids. This may be insignificant at first, but after a number of years this overproduction will probably lead to the development of an ulcer. Similar comparisons can be made with all the other organs and nerves within the body.

Many people have subluxations that they don't know about. This is because subluxations are not painful, and you cannot tell if you have one unless you have your spine examined. Thus the importance of regular spinal checks.

Knowing that your spinal bones are in proper alignment with no nerve interference gives you peace of mind as well as the benefits of maximum nerve supply to all of the organs of your body.

AMAZING ISN'T IT?

DO YOU KNOW YOUR STOMACH?

One of the great mysteries of your body is how its innate intelligence is able to produce hydrochloric acid from the stomach... a mineral acid that's so strong, one drop on your hand will raise a painful blister... without harm to your stomach!

The answer, naturally, is that's the way all mankind is created. The cells in your stomach's lining produce millions of tough, tiny flakes of mucus that line its inside walls just like shingles cover the roof of a house. This lining is replaced every five days due to the powerful acid, along with two other chemicals, pepsin and rennin which are necessary to help break down the food you eat into a consistency that your intestine can digest.

The stomach can hold a little over a quart of food, although this capacity varies among different people. Primitive people were able to gorge themselves with enormous amounts of food because they were never sure when they'd eat again. But don't try it... you'd be mighty uncomfortable.

Every day your stomach produces as much as 2½ quarts of gastric juices to facilitate digestion. You digest a meal in one to seven hours, depending on what and how much you eat. When your stomach is empty, its muscles contract rhythmically. These are the "hunger pangs" you feel. When it's full, it contracts strongly three times per minute. This helps break up the food and push it toward a valve at the lower end of your stomach called the pylorus.

Worries, or hard exercise right after eating slow down your digestion. If it slowed down too much, bacteria and the intestinal flora will cause the food to ferment. This makes you uncomfortable. Anger turns your stomach a fiery red and makes it churn vigorously... Fright makes it lie still, giving you a feeling of "butterflies in your stomach".

In 70 years, your stomach will produce about 60,000 quarts of digestive juice... It will digest about 40 tons of food! You can help your stomach to do its work efficiently by eating properly and making sure the nerve supply to your stomach is free from vertebral subluxations.

Did you know that all of these amazing functions of your stomach are going on right now without you even noticing them? You don't have to know exactly how much gastric juice or hydrochloric acid to produce in order to digest the food you had for breakfast this morning...

It is controlled directly by the innate intelligence of your body through the use of your brain and your nerve system. Of course, if you have vertebral subluxations blocking the mental impulses traveling through your nerve system, you could develop malfunction with your stomach. This could lead to an over-production of hydrochloric acid and given time, could irritate the lining of your stomach and produce an ulcer or even cancer.

The Straight Chiropractor, by correcting vertebral subluxations, ensures a proper nerve supply to your stomach and all the parts of your body. The result is a better expression of your innate potential.

AMAZING ISN'T IT?

THE RESPIRATORY SYSTEM
DO YOU KNOW YOUR LUNGS?

Every day your body uses about 90 gallons of pure oxygen. To separate this gas from the air, the innate intelligence of the body uses your lungs.

The lungs contain half of a billion (500 million) tiny air sacs with a surface area of 50 to 60 square miles! The walls of the sacs and of the blood vessels that wind around and around each one are one cell thick. Molecules of oxygen leave the air in the sacs and pass right through these two one-cell walls into your blood. At the same time, molecules of carbon dioxide gas (which your body must get rid of) go from your blood into the air sacs and are exhaled with your breath. This process is called diffusion.

With every breath you inhale, you breathe in 10^{22} physical atoms which will become part of your brain, kidneys, spleen, gallbladder, etc... That's an astronomical number of atoms. Each time you exhale, you breathe out 10^{22} physical atoms also, ridding yourself of parts of your brain, spleen, heart, liver, etc... so, we literally breathe each others' body parts. We are more intimately interconnected than we believe, physiologically and physically at least.

If the air you breathe reached your lungs without being filtered, you wouldn't live very long. Your lungs would quickly become clogged with dust because with every breath you take, you breathe in dust. And that dust is also laden with toxic materials. But to prevent this, you also possess a marvelous filtering system in which tears, mucus, and tiny hairs all play a part.

This system also prevents the lungs from being scorched by hot air, or frozen by cold air. In cold weather the innate intelligence of the body warms the air. In hot weather it cools the air as it passes into your lungs.

Tears flow out through special ducts from your eyes into your nose. They are very important because they help in moistening and purifying the air you breathe. Also, they contain a germ-killing substance called "lysosyme".

Again, we see the importance of maintaining a good nerve supply to the lungs, because the innate intelligence of the body uses the brain and the nerve system to control and coordinate the respiratory system. If the lungs do not receive the proper amount of energy from the brain, they will not function properly and eventually may develop symptoms (like rapid breathing, slow breathing, painful breathing) and diseases (like asthma, tuberculosis, upper respiratory infection, bronchitis, cancer).

The Straight Chiropractor corrects vertebral subluxations of the nerve system to insure better expression of your innate potential, thus allowing the proper amount of energy to flow from the brain to your respiratory system and all parts of your body.

AMAZING ISN'T IT?

DO YOU KNOW YOUR MUSCLES?

Muscles are like strong steel cables. Each muscle is made up of long, thin cells wrapped in small bundles. The small bundles make up larger bundles and the larger bundles make a muscle.

You have three kinds of muscles:

1-Voluntary (or striped). They move when you want them to.

2-Smooth. They do their work without you directing them (for example, those in your stomach).

3-Heart muscle. It has more reserve power than other muscles and is made of cells shaped like tiny planks.

There are more than 800 muscles in your body! Many muscles work together in teams... More than 200 muscles are working together in order for a man to lift dumb-bells... 31 are used in his face as he strains and clenches his jaw!

Some muscles have red and white fibers. The red fibers work more slowly than the white ones, but can work for a longer time. The white fibers provide your burst of speed. A hummingbird's wing muscles move more than 100 times per second! Even when you aren't moving, dozens of your muscles are working. For example, those in your neck hold your head erect. When you doze off, your neck muscles relax.

Muscles use oxygen, sugars, and fatty acids as fuel. They give off heat to keep you warm. When you run fast they give off so much heat that you perspire to cool off. In cold weather your muscles "shiver" to generate more heat. As muscles work, they use lots of fuel from the blood. You breathe harder and your heart pumps faster to supply more oxygen and remove the waste, but after a time, the blood can't keep it up. You feel tired and must rest until the fuel is replaced in your muscles and all the waste is carried away. Unless you use you muscles regularly and have a good nerve supply to them, they become weak. Do some physical work, exercise each day and get your nerve system free from vertebral subluxations to keep fit.

We cannot stress enough the importance of a good nerve supply, especially when it concerns your muscles. If muscles do not receive the proper quantity and quality of mental impulses they may eventually atrophy, become spastic, tremble or even paralyze.

The Straight Chiropractor corrects vertebral subluxations which interfere with the proper flow of nerve energy. This allows a better expression of the innate potential of the body, thus insuring the muscles and all the parts of your body to function properly.

AMAZING ISN'T IT?

DO YOU KNOW YOUR CELLS?

Like every other living thing, you began your life as one cell. This single cell came about from the egg of your mother and the sperm of your father and it grew, divided and multiplied itself into the quadrillions of cells that are you.

Your cells are of many shapes and sizes. Four thousand cells of the same size laid side by side would make a row only one inch long! When you were a baby you grew very fast because your cells were multiplying rapidly. Gradually your rate of growth slowed down. Between 9 and 11 years of age you began to spurt up again for three to four years. After 20, you grow heavier but no taller.

Girls usually grow faster than boys until they are around 15, then they slow down while boys keep on growing. Boys and girls for many generations have been growing in size. Most of you today are taller than knights of old.

Your cells take in food and oxygen and give off waste. They have the ability to excrete, be productive and reproduce themselves. Cells that have completed their life cycle are replaced by new cells... this process is called regeneration. Basically every year, your body renews itself. For example, heart cells live about 90 days. Red blood cells, 120 days. Liver cells, 300 days. Stomach lining cells, 5 days. Even the DNA which contains millions of years of genetic information is different every 6 weeks. The innate intelligence of the body renews our cells at the rate of 500 million per day. We actually change our bodies more rapidly than we change our clothes.

But new cells don't mean healthy cells. In order for the innate intelligence of the body to regenerate new, healthy cells, the body must be free from vertebral subluxations since the brain and the nerve system coordinate all the cells of your body. Therefore, it is vitally important to check if your body has any vertebral subluxations which interfere with the normal flow of mental impulses. If you do not, chances are that your body will regenerate abnormal cells and when you have many abnormal cells in an organ or gland, it may, over time, malfunction and deteriorate.

When vertebral subluxations are corrected, the natural process of cellular replacement allows your body to express more of its innate potential.

AMAZING ISN'T IT?

IS IT DIVISION OR MULTIPLICATION?

Without cell division, further tissue growth would be prevented by the size limitation of single cells. In the process of cell division called mitosis, each new daughter cell grows to the size of the parent. These new cells, more than 200 million are created in your body every minute, replacing injured and worn out cells. Old, damaged cells self-destruct by releasing a powerful enzyme that digests the cell from within. The innate intelligence of the body controls all of these functions using the central nerve system as its tool to send messages and instructions.

The time it takes a cell to move through the complete cycle, from growth to division, varies enormously. It may take as little as a few hours, or it may last as long as the body lives. Some skin cells live about 8 hours, cells that line the intestine about 1½ days, heart cells about 90 days, red blood cells about 120 days, while undamaged muscle and nerve cells last a lifetime.

AMAZING ISN'T IT?

WHAT ARE THE SECRETS OF THE HUMAN CELL?

Every human being begins life as a single cell, a fertilized egg, and by the time he reached adulthood, his body consists of some 40,000 trillion cells. The cell is the fundamental component of all living things. As cells deteriorate, people age, and as cells malfunction their human performance decreases. If cellular organization was better understood, people might live longer and perform better throughout their entire lifetime.

Scientists discovered three centuries ago that living things contain cells, but only in the last six decades have they begun to piece together the puzzle of how cells operate. They know a few fundamental things: every single adult cell (except ova and sperm) contains the same set of genes as the original cell. Still, cells come in all shapes, sizes and functions: slim nerve cells, more than three feet long and about $\frac{1}{40,000}$th of an inch wide, transmit impulses between the body-cells and the brain cells while red blood cells, sculpted like poker chips and $\frac{3}{10,000}$th of an inch in diameter, carry life giving oxygen around the body. However, researchers remain baffled by the innate intelligence of the body using chemical mechanisms that enable particular genes in different cells to switch themselves on and off and perform differently in varying circumstances.

Each of those quadrillion cells functions like a walled city. Power plants generate the cells' energy. Factories produce proteins, vital units of chemical commerce. Complex transportation systems guide specific chemicals from point to point within the cell and beyond. Sentries at the barricades control the export and import markets, and monitor the outside world for signs of danger. Disciplined biological armies stand ready to grapple with invaders. A centralized genetic government maintain order. An innate intelligence directs some trillion operations every moment.

However, just like political institutions, cells occasionally go wrong. Recycling systems can break down, overloading the cells with their own toxic garbage. Confused by erroneous information, internal factories can add so many chemicals to an already abundant supply that they eventually flood the whole body. A breakdown in communication between the nuclei of cells and their outer borders can produce unrestricted growth of tissues. An interference to the nerve system prevents the body from expressing its own innate potential thus permitting any of the above mishaps to occur and more. Even if they operate smoothly, normal cells eventually succumb to old age... the process of biological decay that alters the cells and kills the organisms which form the basic units.

The human cell and its organelles or interior parts still guard many secrets.

Scientists want to know most of all what mechanism causes the process known as "cell regulation", why certain cells in the pancreas produce insulin, others supply muscles with their power and still others serve the thousands of remaining bodily needs. How do the outer skins or membranes of the cell cooperate with the genes to repel invaders while allowing necessary chemicals and food supplies to move in and out? What controls how genes transmit their instructions for creating vital chemicals in the cells' "factories" or ribosomes?

Each answer seems to pose a new, more complex question about the cell. It seems to be an infinite field. We are just at the beginning, but then, we will always be at the beginning. If anything is certain in the minute and mysterious world of cells, it is that the human cell will never surrender all of its secrets to the human mind. Only the innate intelligence of the body knows everything there is to know about the human cell, and that is enough for us to continue on the course of life.

AMAZING ISN'T IT?

DO YOU KNOW YOUR BODY CHEMISTRY?

We normally think of the human environment in terms of weather and seasons, cities and towns, families and friends. But the true environment is none of these things. Instead, it is a solution of warm salt water inside the body containing sodium, calcium and potassium, magnesium and phosphate, and a number of other ingredients. This solution bathes and nourishes every cell in the human body, and so forms their immediate and vital environment, which is under the direct control of the innate intelligence of the body.

About 70% of the body's weight is water and over half of it is contained inside the cells themselves. Most of the remainder is a bath which surrounds the cells. A fraction of it forms the liquid part of the blood. As the blood courses through the tiny capillaries that pass close to every cell, some of the liquid diffuses, carrying nutrients into the cellular bath to provide the materials cells need for life. At the same time a bit of the bath containing waste products of the cells is drawn out into the bloodstream and goes to the kidneys, where it is purified.

The composition of this cellular bath is so important that most of the major organs of the body mainly concern themselves with insuring the proper proportion of its ingredients, among them the breathing lungs, the pumping heart and filtering kidneys and great areas of the lower brain.

The need for all of this precise regulation is illustrated by the alarming disturbances which can result (particularly in the immune system) if only one of these ingredients moves out of bounds. The innate intelligence of the body uses the brain stem and nerve system to regulate body chemistry. When vertebral subluxations interfere with proper transmission of mental impulses within the nerve system of the body, regulation of body chemistry becomes out of balance.

The Straight Chiropractor corrects vertebral subluxations allowing the body to better express its innate potential. As a result the body's nerve system can detect imbalances so quickly that they are actually corrected as they occur. It does this through an ingenious collection of monitors and sensing devices and it is the interrelation and integration of all these factors (nerve impulses, sensitive monitors, receptors, and regulating organs) that produce the most precise and subtle balance of your body chemistry so necessary in order for your body to perform properly.

AMAZING ISN'T IT?

THINKING OF GOING SOUTH?

On a moonlit night at Ascension Island, a green sea turtle wades ashore after eight weeks of battling South Atlantic currents on a 1,300 mile odyssey from Brazil. The giant turtle lumbers to the stretch of beach where she was born, lays her eggs three feet deep in the sand, and a few hours later begins to paddle back to South America. In two months, the hatchlings will feel the same biological urge to migrate, and they will start their own journey to Brazil. Sometime between 8 and 35 years later, this new generation will return to Ascension, continuing a cycle that has existed for centuries.

Animal migration remains one of the great puzzles of nature, but the last five years have brought an unprecedented scientific quest to understand it. Biologists want to know how blackpoll warblers, songbirds that live in Alaska and weigh less than one ounce, can navigate across Canada to the Maritime Provinces and New England every autumn, then fly nonstop to South America, 2,400 miles away. Scientists hope to learn how monarch butterflies flutter 2,000 miles every September from New England to a single grove of trees on a Mexican mountain. And they are studying how fish find their natal streams 1,200 miles across featureless oceans.

Of course to find out that homing pigeons possess magnetic compasses within themselves, that salmon "smell their way home" a navigation cue to get home and that some butterflies can use the sun and might even hear distinctive sounds of atmospheric pressure to find out where to go, seems to be very stimulating and aesthetically irresistible. However, we should realize that whatever controls our universe is highly organized and controls us also, since we are a part of our universe. Doesn't it make you wonder about yourself in the presence of such wisdom and power?

The same mechanisms at work in the above wonders (salmon, birds, turtles, butterflies) are at work within us. For example: In the male of our species, with each ejaculation are hundreds of thousands of sperm racing to meet one tiny female egg. A journey unexplained by science, the secret remaining locked within the life processes of these living creatures, the sperm. How do the sperm know "where to go" in this somewhat dark vaginal and uterine environment? Do they merge left or right? With amazing accuracy and infallible organization they travel toward the egg floating within the fertile womb. As science knows, in each woman the receptive egg rests one month in her left fallopian tube and the next month in her right one. Again we see that the innate intelligence of the body needs no help in the procreating process, just no interference.

The Straight Chiropractor corrects interferences to the nerve system called vertebral subluxations. This allows the body to express more of its innate potential thereby knowing exactly what to do or not to do at any given moment.

AMAZING ISN'T IT?

IS SCIENCE GOOD OR BAD?

A few moral philosophers who have begun to question whether advancement or objective knowledge is an absolute good, have begun to question whether even our greatest achievements do indeed constitute progress. And other thoughtful persons have somewhat lost confidence in the value of the scientific endeavor, not because they hold pure science or scientists in any less esteem, but because their faith that scientific research will inevitably yield public benefit has been shaken by recent revelations of unpredicted negative impacts of science-based technologies.

Although scientists are frequently disturbed about the level of scientific literacy of the general public and worried about the two cultures among educated folk, the lives of billions of persons worldwide have been immeasurably enriched by some small knowledge of science.

Over the course of their lives men and women coped with deprivation, disease and insufficiency by trying to determine the causes and cures of their wants for things they lacked yet desired. They did this by replacing belief with knowledge through a pursuit called science.

Thus science was born when, in response to needs and wants, substance was given to flashes of inner intuition by those who may be said to have been the first to practice the art of scientific inquiry and proof. Science is, in a way, a human activity which was first practiced as an art. Its power was soon recognized and begun to be used not only to give reality to intuitive innate ideas but as a way of consciously posing questions.

Over the course of time, people have learned to treat many of the diseases and pestilences that prevailed in the past, and have changed their life by trying to bring under control the factors arising outside their own bodies. But unfortunately this has failed as we see our system of health care being dismantled little by little. The main reason of our failure to maintain and improve our health resides mostly in that disease, which still plagues people, arises from internal rather than external causes.

As people turn their attention inward in an effort to understand nature and its influence within themselves, they come face to face with an order of complexity far greater than any they have tried to encompass heretofore. It would not help to emphasize this complexity here, since we have done it so many times before. However, we would prefer to try to simplify the problem by indicating the nature of the basic relationships of true science allowing us to realize that the complex internal machinery required to carry on the particular function of each specialized cell of the human body must be under precise intelligent control.

Our greatest challenge is to maximize the degree of understanding, to share as widely as possible the scientist's aesthetic pleasure in the workings of nature.

This is what this book is all about!

AMAZING ISN'T IT?

ARE MICROBES AND GERMS GOOD FOR YOU?

In common usage, the meaning of the word "nature" is extremely limited. It does not refer to the earth as shaped by cosmic forces, but almost exclusively to the living forms on which people depend and to the earth's atmosphere and surface. The interdependence between human beings and the other forms of life is so complete that the word nature usually has biological connotations, even when referring to inanimate substances. In practice, we do not live on the planet earth but with the life it harbors and within the environment that life creates.

For example, the oxygen we breathe is a product of life. Oxygen was being released into the atmosphere in a free form by primitive organisms that lived more than two billion years ago according to scientific historians. It is still being produced by most members of the plant kingdom, by the microscopic algae of ocean plankton as well as by the most gigantic trees. Microbes and plants are thus absolutely necessary for the existence of animals and human beings, not only because they produce food but also because they literally create a breathable atmosphere.

Like the atmosphere, the present surface of the earth is also apart of the creation of life. Everywhere, under natural conditions, the topsoil is alive with insects, grubs, earthworms, etc, transforming it chemically and physically. This is true whether the soil supports forests, prairies, tundra, grasslands, farmlands, gardens or parks. Organic gardeners have legitimate scientific reasons to claim that earthworms contribute as much as fertilizers to the fertility of the soil. In fact, the microbial forms of life which are invisible to the naked eye are at least as important as earthworms and insects. Every speck of humus contains billions of living germs, belonging to countless different varieties, each specialized in the decomposition and transformation of one or another type of organic debris derived from animals, plants, or other types of microbes. The expert can often detect the activities of germs in the soil simply by handling and smelling it when warm and humid weather increases the intensity of microbial life. Surprising as it may seem, germs account for a large percentage of the total mass of living matter on the earth.

Experience shows that under usual conditions the remnants of animals and plants do not accumulate in nature. Very rapidly they are consumed by germs and thereby taken through a chain of chemical alterations which break them down step by step into simpler compounds. The germs themselves eventually die, and their bodies are also transformed by microbial action. In this manner the constituents of all living things are returned to nature after death to be recycled. Reduced to simpler forms, they are available for the creation of new microbial and plant life, which is eventually consumed by animals and human beings. Microbes and germs thus constitute indispensable links in the chain that binds inanimate matter of life.

The power that animates the living world, including us, needs no help, just no interference.

AMAZING ISN'T IT?

WHAT ARE SOME OF THE RESIDENTS OF THE BODY?

We live in a world dense with microbes: bacteria, viruses and fungi abound in the air, water, and soil, and on the living things around us. Most of these organisms have little interest in the human species. However, a specialized few find the human body an inviting habitat: warm, protected, and well stocked with nutrients. Some settle in the nose and ears, some on the skin and in the intestinal tract.

Usually, we live in harmony with these microscopic residents. Most stay on the body's surfaces. Yet, under certain conditions, when we are malnourished, exhausted, injured, or under stress causing subluxations, resident organisms and other microbes may invade and multiply in our tissues, or set forth in the bloodstream, traveling to all parts of the body. If unchallenged, they can cause serious, even fatal afflictions.

Considering the number of potential interlopers, disease occurs very rarely. This is no accident. Nearly every human possesses a sophisticated and efficient system that works 24 hours a day in every part of the body to ensure good health. Known as the immune system, which is controlled by the innate intelligence of the body, this network of cells and organs responds almost instantaneously to the presence of any disease-causing intruder, mustering its forces to halt the progress of a polio virus or to thwart the efforts of a meningococcus bacterium.

We rely on this powerful system not just to repel disease-causing microbes, but to keep house inside the body. Good health depends on order and consistency among body cells, tissues and organs. The innate intelligence through the immune system preserves this state of balance by removing dead or damaged cells and by seeking out and eliminating wayward or mutant cells.

AMAZING ISN'T IT?

DO OUR BODIES HAVE A SANITATION CREW?

As we breathe, sometimes small particles of bacteria may make it deep down the respiratory tract, landing on the walls of the trachea and bronchial tubes. Special cells and glands in the membranes that line these walls secrete a slightly sticky fluid, mucus, which traps and holds dirt, debris, and microorganisms. Tiny hairlike projections called cilia, which carpet the membrane, then sweep the material away from the surface. With rapid, forceful strokes, the cillia push the mucus and debris out of the passage at the rate of about an inch a minute. This escalator of cilia removes nearly all foreign material to a part of the throat near the mouth called the oropharynx, where it can be coughed out, or swallowed and eventually eliminated from the digestive tract with other wastes. Heavy smoking can paralyze the action of cilia and thus lower the smoker's resistance to respiratory infections.

Sometimes we inhale particles that excite sensitive receptors in the nose, triggering a sneeze, or in the air passages beyond the nose, provoking a cough. The rush of air produced by a cough moves at a speed approaching 600 miles per hour, propelling debris and mucus up and out of the respiratory tract.

Microbes that enter the body by way of the mouth confront waves of saliva loaded with the enzyme lysozyme and other microbe-killing substances. Lysozyme, which also occurs in tears and nasal secretions, destroys bacteria by digesting their cell walls.

Microbes that avoid the protective agents in the mouth find their way to the stomach. There most succumb to the powerful acid secreted by cells in the stomach lining. Others get caught in the sticky mucus that coats stomach and intestines. The wavelike motion known as peristalsis, which moves food through the digestive tract, pushes the mucus and microbes from the body under the direction of its innate intelligence.

AMAZING ISN'T IT?

DO YOU KNOW YOUR SPECIAL SENSES?

All the senses: vision, hearing, smell, taste, touch originate in organs called receptors, specialized to continually instruct the brain about the body's condition and environment. Sense receptors respond to stimuli in the environment by initiating a chain of electrochemical nerve impulses that travel on particular neuronal pathways to regions of the brain that analyze the signals and induce any part of the body.

Usually we filter out 99% of the sights, sounds, and other sensations around us because they do not seem significant or threatening. If we did not, the sensory overload would drive us crazy. Yet, we can call to our consciousness far more sensory data than we originally identify. Any one of us could tabulate a "whole sense" catalog of our surroundings at a hypothetical moment. Tune in on all the sensations around you, the hum of a fan, the liquid twitter of the mockingbird on the fence outside the window, the whir of the neighbor's well-tuned car, the perfume of honeysuckle from the yard, the roughness of the sandals on your bare feet, the blue, red, beige lozenges of the Oriental rug, the corner of a page in your book, its crispness remembered by your fingertips... the pressure of the chair that supports you... soft voices from another room.

Helen Keller was stricken blind and deaf as an infant, isolated from the world and from her fellow human beings. But during childhood the sensitive receptors in her fingertips put her in touch with the world. By feeling, she studied objects, nature, people and experiences the thoughts and emotions that made her a human being. As a girl of 14, she sat at the side of Samuel Clemens as her fingers "read from his lips" the stories he told.

AMAZING ISN'T IT?

DOES IT HURT?

Pain is a sensation we seldom get used to. Pain is an alarm that warns of tissue injury. The several million free nerve endings are our pain receptors, and the more we get hit, the more it hurts. Some pains prick, some burn, some ache. A prickling sensation travels to the brain the fastest, up to 98 feet per second, and locates its source more precisely in the skin's outer layer. A signal of burning pain or of an ache travels more slowly, no more than about six and a half feet per second; originates deeper in the skin; or seems to come from a more diffused, generalizes site, such as the neck or back. Thus, we feel a sharp prickling pain first (from a wasp sting for instance), then the slow burn. The simplest pain response is a sharp reflex that travels only to the spinal cord- an even speedier means of protection when it is necessary to snatch back one's hand from a frying pan.

Our sensory apparatus, with the autonomic nervous system, monitors functions inside the body. Digestion proceeds, blood circulates, lungs expand and contract. We are seldom conscious of these messages.

AMAZING ISN'T IT?

WHY DO WE SAY OUCH?!

About 17 inches long, up to three-quarters of an inch thick, and as flexible as a rubber hose, the spinal cord provides the main link between the brain and the rest of the body. Thirty-one pairs of spinal nerves containing hundreds of thousands of individual nerve fibers emerge through holes in the spinal cord's bony protector, the spinal column. Thousands more fibers project from the bottom of the spinal cord in a cluster called the cauda equina, or horse's tail before they, too, exit through the spinal column.

Inside the spinal cord, millions of nerve cell bodies in the grey matter process sensory and motor input and handle automatic reflex actions. Touch a hot stove, and your hand jerks back instantly because of a spinal cord command. Conscious reactions occur when the spinal cord relays messages to and from the brain via nerve fibers in the white matter. You feel pain and know you have burned fingers because a report was sent to your brain by way of the spinal cord as the spinal cord mediated a reflex action in your muscles.

AMAZING ISN'T IT?

IS IT YOURS OR MINE?

Can you touch your fingertips to each other behind your back? Can you close your eyes and find your feet? Can you walk in a straight line? You probably can. The reason is that our bodies possess a sense sometimes called kinesthetic (from the Greek for "perception of motion"), and are served by their own proprioceptors. (Proprio' comes from Latin "for ones own") The information that some of the proprioceptors send to, the brain creates some of the most fundamental components of our sense of self. Few of us go through the day giving close attention to what each part of our body is doing and where it is. Yet we are aware, subliminally, and continually process information from proprioceptors, consciously using it to direct action. Look around at people you know. One may be a piano player, another a roller skater, another a champion runner. Proprioceptors are at work here, as they are in the performance of daily chores like washing dishes and driving a car.

Pacinian corpuscles and other receptors in the joints, ligaments, muscles and tendons respond to the stimulation that occurs when we move a joint. Some monitor the rate of movement and the tension of muscles. Others signal our position in space. Still others measure pressure changes... when you turn a steering wheel, then relax your grip, or when a quarterback reaches for the ball, then takes it... and continually tell the brain what is going on. These messages travel very fast and produce varying degrees of coordination.

AMAZING ISN'T IT?

IS THERE TRULY AN ELECTRIC BRAIN?

The infinite wisdom of your body called innate intelligence conceived, manufactured, assembled, coordinated and distributed over 400 trillion tissue cells, each one with a specific function to perform in 280 days. That's amazing!

The first group of cells to differentiate into a system were the brain cells. Your brain is the first organ to appear as your body developed within the womb of your mother.

Your brain sends and receives thousands of signals from your entire body via your nerves every moment of your life, day and night. Your innate intelligence does the decoding and interpretation of these messages. For example: Your brain gets information from 130 millon light receptors in your eye... 100,000 hearing receptors in your ears... 3,000 taste buds in your mouth... 30,000 heat spots, 250,000 cold spots, and 500,000 touch spots on your skin.

When you were born, your brain weighed a pound, or about ⅛th of your body weight. When you are grown it will weigh around three pounds depending upon your stature, body weight, and sex. This is larger in proportion to body size than other creatures of our planet.

Your brain operates by electricity. Each nerve cell in your body generates an amazing voltage for its size. This can be measured by EKG, EEG, and EMG which are instruments using voltmeters as their main components. Each nerve cell passes chemo-electical impulses (also comprised of chemicals) on to the next nerve cell. Your brain cells generate a similar current to send back orders to your muscles and other organs. These chemo-electric impulses flash along your nerves at 393 feet per second, or about 270 miles per hour... so your reactions are mighty fast.

Your innate intelligence usually produces within each nerve cell 2 to 50 impulses per second. But, it can produce up to 2,000 per second. The impulses are all the same, whether they're from your toes, eyes, tongue, or any other part of your body including such organs as the stomach, pancreas, heart, liver, etc... However, since each impulse contains a different code within itself and the innate intelligence makes the decoding and interpretation, the entire process is extremely intelligent and calculated. For this reason, these impulses are called mental impulses.

Some parts of your brain called the medulla oblongata (brain stem) serve as a "center" to relay messages. Some parts control vital processes such as breathing, some do your thinking, and others hold your memories in storage until you call for them, very much like a hard drive.

Of all the systems and organs in the body, the one responsible for the coordination of the rest of the body is the brain and the nerve system. It is the first organ of the body to develop and because of its importance, is protected by the skull and the vertebral column. However, due to physical, emotional, or chemical trauma, the vertebrae can become displaced to a degree sufficient to interfere with the flow of mental impulses. When this happens, disorder and chaos develop within the body.

The Straight Chiropractor corrects these interferences to the nerve system which restore the normal flow of mental impulses. This allows the body to function in a state of order and harmony once again and permits greater expression of its innate potential. Remember that every organ of your body is attached to the one under your hat!

AMAZING ISN'T IT?

DID YOU KNOW?

All authorities unanimously agree that in order to have NORMAL BODY FUNCTIONS we must have adequate, unrestricted, uninterrupted mental impulses flow from the brain, through the nerves, to the tissue cells of the body! Proper nerve supply is essential for expressing one's full innate potential through our human experience. The fact that the nerve system is the master communication system of the body is a settled fact of true science. It has been demonstrated at the University of Rochester, New York by Dr. Finkelstein and his group of scientists that the nerve system and the immune system are one and the same. This gives the nerve system a much more flexible approach to completely control and coordinate all the cells of the human body.

When scientists first discovered this in 1993, they were totally amazed at what they had discovered. The entire scientific community was struck to the core and had to admit that chiropractic was right over 100 years ago and was definitely ahead of its time.

With this discovery, it naturally follows that in good health and ill health the nerve system becomes the regulating force. In good health the flow of mental impulse is normal; we can see, taste, hear, smell, feel and function. By it, we move, breathe, have our being, plan and understand. We mend fractures, repair wounds, grow, adapt, excrete and assimilate. In ill health however, the flow of mental impulse is altered and we cannot perform well any longer. We dramatically understand as well that the absence of mental impulse flow (also called brain waves) indicated death. In other words, through the mental impulse flow from brain to tissue cell and back to the brain, we LIVE.

Health (being 15% of the human experience) is simply the normal, natural, free expression that this mental impulse flow under the perfect control of innate intelligence through the nerve system.

Vertebral subluxations interfere with this mental impulse flow by causing an insult to the nerve system because of the pressure exerted by the vertebrae on the brain stem, the spinal cord or the spinal nerves.

The Straight Chiropractor locates, analyzes and corrects vertebral subluxations by adjusting the spine.

Chiropractic is comprised of more than 30 principles and teaches that when a vertebrae is subluxated (out of its normal alignment, producing nerve interference) it alters the line of communication between brain cell and tissue cell, and the end result is less expression of the innate potential, also called a state of dis-ease (incoordination or malfunction within the body).

Only Chiropractic recognizes and claims the understanding of dis-ease (body malfunction), while all other professions treat effects of dis-ease (symptoms, pain, syndromes, diseases, infection and the like). Chiropractic is scientific in locating and analyzing vertebral subluxations and can duplicate its results. Chiropractic is the art of adjusting specifically the spinal column for the correction of vertebral subluxations. Chiropractic is the philosophy of understanding how to express more of the innate potential within the confines of human experience.

A normal functioning body alone has the inherent ability, perfection, wisdom and capacity for healing and restoration to wholeness. Under the specific care of a Straight Chiropractor, human beings possess the ability to express more of their innate potential.

A person's life should be like a candle, burning with a bright flame to the very end of the wick, and then a short sputtering dimness, a final sputter and finally, darkness. Human beings should enjoy full powers and functions to the very day life terminates, their light as bright as the brightness of the candle before the final sputter.

Chiropractic will help you achieve nobility and dignity for your life.

AMAZING ISN'T IT?

ART

CAN THE WORLD WITHIN GO WRONG?

Imprisoned in the narrowness of our human scale, we are blind to vast reaches of reality. Mysteries lie all around us, even within us, waiting to be revealed by a new way of seeing. Just as a journey to the moon may show us the daintiness of our planet, a venture into the minuscule can be a true voyage of discovery.

An exploration of the human species should properly begin with an exploration of the nerve system, for that great mass of cells and fibers contains the way stations and pathways which determine what is uniquely human in our nature. The nerve system can be regarded as a complex computer. Its essential components are the nerve cells, or neurons. An enormous number of neurons participate in this process we call life. The central nerve system is composed of four major interconnected elements: the cerebrum, the cerebellum, the brain stem and the spinal cord.

The innate intelligence of the body uses the human brain to generate energy which is sent down the spinal cord in impulses going through and over the nerve fibers which consequently nurture the organs, glands and systems of the body.

The nerve system is protected by a column of bones called the vertebral column. Of course, sometimes things can go wrong and the body can begin to perform improperly. Fortunately, the body has so many back-up devices and so much extra capacity that it can take a lot of use and abuse and still balance its oxygen and food, its water and salts, its heat and cold.

Because of the high flexibility of the human vertebral column some of the vertebrae may move out of place causing pressure on the nerve system. When this happens, we say the body has a vertebral subluxation and is not expressing all of its innate potential. This puts the body in a state of dis-ease, meaning a state of malfunction. What the body needs then is a chiropractic adjustment to restore the integrity of the nerve system which will allow the body to return to a state of ease, meaning a state of proper function by expressing more of its own innate potential.

If the body does not get the required adjustment, it can end up with not quite enough or a bit too much energy causing problems in the attempt of balancing its oxygen and food, its water and salts, its heat and cold, in other words, balancing its own chemistry. Given enough time, human performance will decrease which can show up in a multitude of physical, physiological, psychological and even spiritual ways.

Straight Chiropractors provide a program of regular spinal check-ups for entire families and if vertebral subluxations are found in someone, they correct them by means of specific adjustments. The net result is a better expression of the innate intelligence of the body in everyone receiving chiropractic care.

AMAZING ISN'T IT?

AWESOME OR NOT?

From an egg to a unique individual – Until Aristotle in ancient Greece broke open hens' eggs and studied the growth of embryos, almost nothing was known about the beginnings of life. A woman's body began to swell and she felt life stirring within her. Where did the baby come from? What did it look like before birth? The fact that the embryo was formed from both father and mother was recognized even in Aristotle's time but the exact contribution of each parent would be debated for centuries.

In 1653, the English surgeon William Harvey, who also studied chick embryos, wrote "an egg can no more be made without the assistance of the cock, and the hen, than the fruit can be made without the tree's aid". Throughout the Middle Ages and much of the Renaissance, scientists considered each individual as preformed from the very moment of conception. Only about 300 years ago, with the discovery of the microscope, did they begin to discern the facts. The male sperm was seen and described in detail. The egg was carefully examined and seen to have its own structures, not those of the adult. Today's scientists can detect the finest structures of egg and sperm, analyze their chemical content and study the embryo's growth from the first moments of life. All that has been learned, however, only increases the sense of awe with which human beings behold the beginning of life.

AMAZING ISN'T IT?

WHAT IS HEALING?

Taeber's Encyclopedic Medical Dictionary defines healing as a "Process of curing: the restoration of wounded parts". This definition of healing is taught in every medical school in the country and leaves much to be desired. To understand the healing process of the body is to further strengthen our confidence in the body and its innate intelligence.

Many people are under the mistaken impression that their doctor healed or cured them. Whether they are medical doctors, osteopathic doctors, or chiropractic doctors, people believe they cured them. Doctors sometimes take credit for effecting a cure. Perhaps this is due to the ego of the human being, however it shows a complete lack of understanding of the healing process, because the idea that a doctor cures anybody is absurd.

Many people will believe that a medication or surgery or an adjustment cured them. Medication can do only one of two things: stimulate a part of the body to work faster or depress a part to work slower, that's all! These are stimulants and depressants called by various names. Not one drug can heal a person. Surgery does not heal anyone either. It merely cuts out a diseased part and imposes the lack of that part on the entire body permanently. Now the body has to try to function with missing something it needed to be performing properly. The body is now in a state of permanent diminished performance which is a lack of health permanently. An adjustment does not cure either but simply allows the correction of a vertebral subluxation which was interfering with the normal quantity and quality flow of mental impulses. When this is accomplished it allows the body to function normally thereby replacing its own cells normally, which in turn causes healing to occur. My point is that it is the innate intelligence of the body that can heal the body as long as there is no interference and is not limited by the matter of the body which it controls.

Let me put it this way: cells are constantly created by the innate intelligence of the body to take the place of the cells that are dying. Cells live only so long. For example, red blood cells live about 120 days, heart cells about 90 days, liver cells about 300 days, stomach lining cells about 5 days, etc. The life expectancy of the cell occurs regardless of whether the cell is sick or not. So why bother try to heal sick cells? Let them die! But make sure that the cells replacing the cells that died are healthier than the ones that just died, otherwise your body will not heal. This is how the healing process occurs, by the creation of new living tissue to take place of the one that has been destroyed.

When you cut your finger you destroy billions of cells. The innate intelligence of the body will heal that cut by creating new cells to take the place of those that have been destroyed. No drugs in the world will heal that cut. The same is true for a sick part. No drugs will heal a sick cell. Tell me what would happen over time to a healthy body if you would pump drugs inside of it? It would get sick. Then, explain how a sick body can become healthy if you pump drugs into it. Nobody has ever been able to explain that to me. By the way, even the body does not have to heal a sick cell. All the body has to do is replace the sick cell with a new healthy cell. This is the way healing takes place within the body. In order for somebody or something to heal they or it must be able to create living tissue.

People have not yet been able to create living tissue out of nothing and it is doubtful that they will ever be able to do so. Only the innate intelligence of the body can do that. We must mention here that in order for a body to be able to create new healthy living tissue it must not have any vertebral subluxations to its nerve system, so it can better express its own innate potential.

The Straight Chiropractor corrects vertebral subluxations and insures better expression of the body's own innate potential thereby allowing normal cells' replacement within the body. This is the Straight Chiropractor's role in the healing process, to make sure that the new tissue is created with 100% of its life energy so that it can be healthy and stay that way.

AMAZING ISN'T IT?

DO YOU WANT TO KNOW MORE HEALING?

The body will always endeavor to heal itself by creating new tissue. However in some instances, complete healing cannot take place. This occurs when the damage is either very extensive or very severe. In the first instance, when the damage is very extensive, the body may not be able to completely heal itself. Everyone has seen this in the case of a very bad cut. The body will heal itself, but it may not be complete. The body can only heal using the material it has to work with. Even if the body does not have enough material with which to produce "body cement" to seal off the wound as best as it can, the innate intelligence of the body is always working for the best interest of the body.

We call this "body cement" scar tissue. In the sense of creating new tissue the body has not completely healed the cut because scar tissue is not living cells, but it is the best possible means in this situation. If it is possible, as time goes on, the innate intelligence of the body will be able to grow new tissue and eventually the scar will grow fainter and fainter. Perhaps, if the damage is very extensive, new tissue will never be created and the person will have the scar forever.

In the second instance, if the damage is very severe, the body will quickly produce scar tissue as an emergency measure to keep the person alive. Scar tissue can be made more quickly than living cells. This often occurs in the person with an acute heart attack. Because of the great amount of scar tissue, the person may never be able to lead an active life again. Scar tissue cannot do the job of the normal healthy living cells. In many cases the innate intelligence of the body, given time and given a good nerve supply, will be able to once again produce the cells necessary for healing to take place. This is why many people who have had severe heart attacks and are under chiropractic care sometimes return to their normal activity. The difference between them and those who are invalids for the rest of their lives is the ability of their bodies to replace scar tissue with living cells. The difference may have been due to a good nerve supply restored by chiropractic adjustments because this allows the body to better express its innate potential.

The living body possesses an innate intelligence that can heal the body. It needs no help from anyone! What it needs is no interference! All the Straight Chiropractor does is to eliminate the nerve interferences called vertebral subluxations to enable the innate intelligence of the body to heal itself.

AMAZING ISN'T IT?

WHAT IS HEALTH?

Health, what is it? It seems to be something people want. Many people spend a lot of time and money searching for it, and all of us miss it if we don't have it. What is this health?

Ask most people, and they'll tell you that health is when you're not feeling sick. If you're not sick, if you're not feeling symptoms, then you're healthy. But is this true? Is health the absence of symptoms?

What is a symptom? What is it that makes us feel we are not well? A symptom is some type of sign that we interpret as being bad for us and this interpretation causes us pain. It is pain that we interpret as a sign of being sick. What happened in our body to cause us pain?

Is it like this – that something begins to go wrong within our body, and instantly we feel pain, and we know we are sick? Or is it this way – that something begins to go wrong just a little, and it is not corrected, and so it builds up, until it reaches the level where it finally causes pain?

Most people believe that symptoms happen at the beginning of a disease. This is completely and totally untrue. Symptoms are not a sign of the beginning of illness, rather, symptoms tell you that something has been wrong for a long time, long enough to build up to the point of causing you pain. Symptoms do not tell you that you just got sick... symptoms tell you that you have been unhealthy for a long time.

So we cannot define health as the absence of symptoms. We need another definition, and in chiropractic, we have one.

Health comes from a Greek word meaning whole. In chiropractic, we know that health equals wholeness. Wholeness has two meanings here. First, wholeness in structure, that all the various parts are present. Second, and most importantly wholeness in function, that each part is coordinated with all the other parts. It is this harmonious wholeness that is health. Health is definitely not "the absence of symptoms." Health is the presence of coordinated proper functioning of all the parts of the body.

In order for your body to function properly, the innate intelligence of the body uses a communication system: the brain and the nerves. By way of the nerves, messages come into the brain, giving feedback about body conditions, and instructions go out from the brain, to keep things working smoothly. This is how the innate intelligence of the body controls and coordinates your functions and keeps you healthy.

The Straight Chiropractor makes sure you are free from any interference to your communication system (brain and nerves) so that the innate intelligence of the body can maintain your body health by allowing it to better express its own potential.

AMAZING ISN'T IT?

VERTEBRAL SUBLUX... WHAT?

A vertebral subluxation is a condition in which nerve control is lost between the brain control centers and the organs by a small displacement of the spinal bones, always diminishing the innate potential of the body.

A vertebral subluxation is an interference to the function of your body forcing you to have less than normal body performance, forcing you to have less than optimal physical, mental and social well-being. It is the most serious interference to the functions of your body that we know of.

A vertebral subluxation causes malfunction of the life support systems in our body, silently eating away at our ability to be all that we could be. It is what the University of Colorado research described as: "The slightest amount of pressure on a spinal nerve root emerging from the spine or at the brain stem which kills the function 60% in a matter of minutes."

It has now been proven that one to three hours of a great deal of pressure causes many of the nerve fibers in the nerve root or brain stem to rupture, producing toxins or poisons which spread to the surrounding tissues. This is the same degree of pressure Straight Chiropractors find in the average person's spine. The poisons in turn, are absorbed into the nerves, bones, ligaments, spinal discs, muscles and other supportive tissues of the spine, progressively and relentlessly destroying them throughout a lifetime. Although a vertebral subluxation may not be felt immediately, its effects are relentless and progressive.

What does it mean to a Straight Chiropractor? It means that he does not look for, nor is he interested in symptoms or signs in determining what he has to do. It means that the vertebral subluxation must be corrected as soon as possible after it occurs.

By attempting to make correction of vertebral subluxations available to everyone throughout the world, the Straight Chiropractor hopes not only to encourage our individual self improvement but also to facilitate the intelligent use of our environment.

AMAZING ISN'T IT?

PRACTICE

WHEN IS A PERSON TOO OLD TO BE UNDER REGULAR CHIROPRACTIC CARE?

No one is ever too old to start regular chiropractic care. Since expressing more of your innate potential is your birthright as well as the only effect of chiropractic care, it should be your lifetime priority! So in this respect one is never too old (or too young) to care to be the best one can be.

In point of fact, we have known people aged 95-102 years to be under regular chiropractic care.

The aging process is a certain fact of life as you no doubt realize: it is unavoidable. However, isn't it amazing that some people well on in years do not "look their age", and indeed, seem to have more energy than their younger counterparts?

This is not a quirk or a rarity; neither should it be surprising. Obviously, if your body is working right, it will have a better supply of energy than if it is not working right.

One of the good results of expressing more of your innate potential is adaptation. Only if your body is able to adapt to its environment (heat, cold, pollen, viruses, bacteria, etc...), to cope with its surroundings or deal with invading microbes and germs do you have a chance to be the best that you can be physically, emotionally, psychologically, etc... If on the other hand, your body does not adapt easily, you will find yourself in a state of dis-ease (malfunction), and a body in a state of dis-ease is certainly not working right.

To illustrate this, let's suppose it is 90 degrees and you are enjoying the morning sun in your backyard. Your body temperature is maintained by the process of adaptation at 98.6 degrees. Adaptation is controlled by the innate intelligence of your body through your nerve system. Suddenly a swift wind blows some clouds over the area and the temperature drops to 76 degrees in a matter of minutes. With the outdoor drop in temperature of 14 degrees, what would be your body temperature? 98.6 degrees of course! Why? Because your body has the ability to adapt according to its own need.

Your body also adapts to germs, viruses, and bacteria. A common example of this is the flu. There are many people who get the flu frequently and never seem to get rid of it; while others have the flu for only a few hours. The virus is in the air and we are all breathing the same air aren't we? Then why are there some people who "don't seem to get rid of it?". Certainly those who get rid of the flu quickly show a better adaptation.

Antibodies are always present within your body. Anybody with a vertebral subluxation will not adapt properly thus increasing their likelihood to malfunction (dis-ease) and will not manufacture the proper kind or correct amount of antibodies. But if your body is functioning without interference to its nerve system, you will adapt normally and consistently and you will then be truly the best you can be.

Be aware that you cannot feel vertebral subluxations and the only way to properly care for your body's adaptation is to see a Straight Chiropractor regularly.

As you can see, at any age, regular chiropractic care adds years to life and life to years.

AMAZING ISN'T IT?

WHAT IS THE COOPERATIVE FEE SYSTEM?

Chiropractic's approach to human performance is NEW and so it is fitting for it to employ a NEW and unique approach to render this service to the public. The cooperative chiropractic office fits the bill. Its purpose is simply to break down the many barriers that prohibit both the providing of superior service and the availability of that service to everyone interested in expressing more of their innate potential.

The job of the Straight Chiropractor is to properly locate, analyze and correct vertebral subluxations, the most terrifying interference to normal body function. To qualify as a patient, it is necessary 1: to be alive, 2: to have a nerve system, 3: to have a spine. In essence, everyone needs regular chiropractic care, since specific adjustments of the spine liberate the life-force energy to be conveyed to all body parts through the nerve system. For when the bones of the spine (vertebra) are slightly displaced from their normal position, they interfere with and inhibit the nerve system causing the body to express less of its innate potential. This in turn creates malfunction within the body and causes cells of the body to lose their ability to excrete properly, to be productive and to reproduce themselves normally. Given time this situation allows the human performance of the body to decrease. Eventually it leads to problems of all kinds, physically, emotionally, psychologically, and spiritually. The entire human performance is affected negatively. Those specific chiropractic adjustments restore the integrity of the nerve system and permit the body to regain and maintain proper function, which in turn allows a better expression of the body's own innate potential. Then the body can recreate itself normally once again increasing human performance and healing completely.

Some barriers that need to be removed for this NEW approach to be effectively workable are 1: prior erroneous notions of human performance, 2: the cost of continuous care. What the cooperative system is designed to do is to transform the doctor/patient/client member relationship from one of mystery and expense to one of mutual understanding and cooperation. It affords us all a unique opportunity to learn more about the life principles of human performance, have access to the best professional care possible and be responsible financially with dignity and honesty for that which is our birthright: a maximum expression of our innate potential.

There are certain responsibilities that are attached to this affordable fee system and that's why it's called a cooperative system. When one understands the vertebral subluxation and its tragic effect on people's lives, one has the moral responsibility to inform others about the vertebral subluxation and refer them to a Straight Chiropractor to hear the chiropractic story. A cooperative office is dependent on a large volume of patients, clients and members in order to thrive and provide its services to its community. To refrain from this responsibility is to let other people be doomed to a life less fulfilling at every level of the human experience.

In summary, to qualify to be a member of a cooperative office, you must 1: bring yourself and your family for weekly chiropractic check-ups, 2: attend the orientations, lectures, classes, workshops and seminars offered, 3: share chiropractic with others. You then become a part of the "informed minority" pressed upon to spread the chiropractic message to the uninformed majority. Tell everyone that chiropractic fosters a better expression of the body's own innate potential, that is improves human performance at all levels of the human experience by correcting vertebral subluxations by means of specific adjustments of the vertebral column. Tell everyone that a cooperative office accepts all persons regardless of their physical or mental condition or their financial ability to pay and that the cooperative fee system is based on the determination of the patient/client/member to pay what is within their means for receiving the chiropractic care they deserve.

AMAZING ISN'T IT?

WHAT IS CELL DIFFERENTIATION?

Cell division alone would create a mass of cells that all look the same within the human body. But some cells need to turn into skin, some into liver, some into brain, and still others into a myriad of other tissues that make up the whole body. To differentiate, the innate intelligence of the body changes the cells structure and appearance and has them assume specialized functions. This process begins with the embryo and, in some cases, continues throughout life. Nerve cells, for example, develop thin strands up to three feet long that transmit stimuli to and from the brain. Their responsibilities are paramount to the proper functioning of the body and for that reason, the vertebral spinal column is comprised of 24 bones that protect these nerve cells.

Oftentimes because of stress, the vertebral column may go out of alignment and that causes pressure on the nerve cells. An interference to the nerve system prevents the body from functioning as it should and causes the resistance of that body to decrease. This is called a subluxation.

As a straight objective chiropractor, I correct subluxations by means of adjustments to allow the body to function without interference.

Going back to differentiation, it results when certain genes within a cell are activated, while others are repressed to prevent the formation of unwanted proteins. Differentiated cells no longer perform many of the functions of other cells, although their nuclei retain all the genes necessary to do so.

AMAZING ISN'T IT?

TOUCH ME, TOUCH ME NOT?

Our bodies possess a continuum of touch receptors that respond to a spectrum of stimuli and sensations, where there may be a fine line between a tickle and a twinge, between pleasure and pain.

When some stimuli are present over a period of time, we adapt to them. We put on clothes every morning and, at first, various receptors send messages to the brain that make us conscious of their weight, texture, and pressure. But before long the messages dwindle and disappear, switched off because continuing stimuli of constant intensity will stop activating the receptors. You can accept an affectionate but heavy cat curled up in your lap, not because the cat gets lighter but because for a time you become oblivious to the pressure. A change must occur to reactivate the receptors. The wristwatch we are so used to that we forget its presence will suddenly attract our attention if the clasp breaks and it threatens to fall off. At the end of the day, receptors will signal the pleasure of removing ties, jackets and tight shoes.

That is why vertebral subluxations (nerve interference or nerve pressure) can go on unnoticed by you for a long period of time. That is the reason for regular chiropractic check-ups.

AMAZING ISN'T IT?

AXLES OR AXONS?

Every few seconds in every day in a lifetime, tens of billions of sensory messages travel as electrochemical impulses along the slender branches of the human nervous system. They make their way to communication headquarters in the central nervous system: the brain and spinal cord. Fifty to one hundred billion nerve cells, or neurons, act as information specialists. Each receive messages on branching arms called dendrites and sends signals via a single nerve fiber, or axon. Axons outside the brain and spinal cord often form cables that bring the brain information from sensory receptors or carry commands to muscles, glands and organs.

Most nerve fibers are sheathed in myelin, which forms a thick outer covering. Myelin acts as an insulator and allows the nerve impulses to move faster. Along large nerve fibers, such as the three foot long branches of the sciatic nerves in the legs, impulses travel up to 290 miles per hour.

Regular adjustment allow the mental impulses to travel without interference. The body then functions better, heals better and demonstrates a higher resistance.

AMAZING ISN'T IT?

DO WE HAVE A RIGHT TO COMPLAIN?

There are moments in everyone's life when it is necessary to stop and search deeply within oneself... to discover what is most important in one's life. Whether we consider what is most important to be a spouse, child, friend, position or money there is something that rises above and ahead of any other priority, namely human performance. Human performance is the primary imperative for the fulfillment of any aspiration in any realm of our lives.

Without effective human performance we are limited in all aspects of our lives. Without proper human performance we become less than we should be for ourselves, our dear ones and society at large. Without maximum human performance we cannot enjoy any marital or love relationship, our children, our friends, our money or any material possession.

Do you remember that last time you were feeling miserable and tried to carry on a romantic moment, or take the kids to the zoo, or conduct a business meeting? Without a doubt, what you remember is not being able to function at your best... your performance was impaired by discomfort, symptoms or disease.

So we see human performance as being the most necessary factor in everyone's life in achieving a state of physical, mental and social well-being. Moreover, the degree to which we are able to enjoy life is directly dependent on the state of our human performance.

It is unfortunate that most of us have been misled into believing that we can take human performance for granted... that we can abuse our bodies and take "care" of them only when exhausted by malfunction which is always causing symptoms and pain as a warning that something is going on that needs our attention. It is ironic but true that the average American spends more energy, time and money caring for their home or car than they do for their own body.

It is our right as free-thinking human beings to tell ourselves: " I don't care about my body and human performance". But it must be remembered that it is the right of the body to complain and breakdown, giving us less than optimum enjoyment of life, resulting in disordered living. If we choose to ignore our bodies and neglect our human performance, then we have no right to complain to anyone but ourselves when the free flow of our lifestyle is interrupted by discomfort and disease.

Human performance is our individual responsibility and we must work at it in order to maintain its maximum potential. The Straight Chiropractor corrects vertebral subluxations which interfere with the proper flow of mental impulses within the nerve system of the body, thereby allowing the body to better express its own innate potential which in turn improves human performance at all levels of the human experience.

AMAZING ISN'T IT?

CAN WE OBSERVE?

Can we observe that:

- Life and health come from within our body, not from a bottle, a pill, a needle or a scalpel?

- The phenomenon of creation did not stop at birth, but is continuously and permanently going on from conception until death?

- New cells are being created every second of our lives within our body?

- The innate inborn power that created our body knows more about how to run that body than the finite, limited knowledge and education of all university graduates put together?

- The nerve system is the system used by the innate inborn power to run, control and coordinate the human body?

- Normal flow of life-energy from the brain along the spinal cord and nerves to the rest of the body means full expression of the body's own innate potential?

- Death by hanging is caused by the neck bones (vertebrae) compressing the nerve system to such an extent that it causes abnormal nerve energy flow from the brain to the rest of the body so seriously that it results in death?

- Any amount of compression to the nerve system caused by a small displacement of a vertebra (back bone) will produce abnormal nerve energy flow from the brain to the rest of the body always resulting in a decrease of human performance and eventually leading to death?

- Unnatural lifestyle, air, water and food pollution, along with physical trauma such as sports injuries, whiplash, falls, fights, strenuous exercises, improper posture, jerks, jolts, slips, exertion and fatigue cause small displacements of vertebrae (back bones), putting pressure upon sensitive nerves, interfering with the natural flow of mental impulses from brain cells to tissue cells, interrupting the flow of energy from the brain to the rest of the body, always resulting in a decrease of human performance and leading eventually to death?

- A NEW approach to human performance enhancement, chiropractic was founded and developed in 1895?

- Chiropractic is not a form of conventional or holistic medicine?

- Chiropractic is strictly and uniquely concerned with the correction of vertebral subluxations which interfere with the transmission of mental impulses between brain and body parts, thereby enhancing human performance by allowing the body to better express its own innate potential?

- The expression of Life and the innate potential of the body is vital to human performance which in turn enhances all levels of the human experience?

- This NEW system has three major aspects, namely: philosophy, art, science... each related to the other, yet dependent upon the philosophy?

- This NEW system of chiropractic is based upon a natural principle concerning human beings and offers a cooperative economical system affordable by all?

- NEW concepts and principles have shaken humanity at a time of revolution and evolution?

- Open-mindedness means investigating NEW principles and ideas?

- Since chiropractic is NEW why not investigate it in its entirety?

- To investigate chiropractic could literally change your life for the better!

AMAZING ISN'T IT?

CAN WE PERCEIVE FULLY WHEN WE LET IT BE?

It is a sad commentary on our civilization that when we speak of the environment it is usually in reference to its undesirable effects. The very word "environment" now evokes the nightmares of industrial and urban life: depletion of natural resources, accumulation of wastes, pollution in all its forms, noise, crowding, regimentation, the thousand devils of ecological crisis. Just as the pilgrim fathers regarded nature around Provincetown Harbor as hideous and full of demons, we fear the world we have created. As a result we are chiefly concerned with the avoidance of dangers and the maintenance of a tolerable state, rather than with the creation of NEW, positive values through the development of environmental and human potentialities.

Thinking about the environment only in such negative terms is not likely to take us far toward the establishment of desirable living conditions. If we limit our efforts to the correction of environmental defects, we shall increasingly behave like hunted beasts taking shelter behind an endless succession of protective devices, each more complex and more costly, less dependable and less comfortable than its predecessors. It is true that the solution to any problem of this magnitude can be found only at a different level from which it was created. Today, we develop afterburners for automobiles to protect us from air pollution and complicated sewage treatments to purify grossly contaminated water. Tomorrow, we shall turn to gas masks and to filters for our water (which exist already). Although technological fixes have some usefulness, they complicate life and eventually decrease its quality. The ecological crisis will continue to increase in severity if we do not develop positive values integrating internal environment (human performance, body ecology, health, human potential) and external environment (the world in which we live, air, water, food, etc...).

Positive values can sometimes be introduced from the outside. More generally, however, they are found in the intimate relationships between human beings and the world in which they live.

A NEW kind of knowledge is needed, moreover, to predict the likely consequences of technological interventions and develop rational guides as substitutes for the adjustments that time used to make possible.

Our restored values must come first and must preside over technology because they provide the basic principles which give aesthetic quality and scientific coherence to the physical structure embodying our social purpose.

Let us stop complaining and being negative toward our society. Let us take positive actions concerning first our personal attitude and second, concerning our taking the responsibilities necessary for gradual ongoing change within ourselves. For only then will we be able to perceive fully... when we let it be.

AMAZING ISN'T IT?

DOES CHANGE TAKE TIME?

Disease is, in reality, life in altered form. Sickness and disease do not happen overnight. It takes years of lack of proper body function and lack of life-energy for symptoms to finally show up.

In other words there are basically three states of ill health. The first is a functional impairment of the body: an organ fails to function properly. This is often impossible to detect and may not be noticed by the patient or the physician. It is an asymptomatic phase; nothing is being felt.

The second state brings definite symptoms of illness. It is the result of malfunction acting upon the body for a length of time. Symptoms are being felt, the patient feels ill.

The third state brings structural changes. The tissue or organ's structure actually changes.

In brief:

1. Malfunction (no symptoms)

2. Definite symptoms

3. Structural changes

At present, people are not concerned about themselves before the second phase has been reached. More often the third phase begins before people start to be concerned about their health.

With the nerve system being the system controlling how our entire body functions, Straight Chiropractors focus their entire energy in maintaining that system free of blockages. In removing interferences to the nerve system, the body is allowed to function properly. This prevents the first, second and third phase from developing.

Straight Chiropractors understand that it makes more sense to maintain proper function than to fight disease. Straight Chiropractors further understand that health lies with proper function rather than with drugs, needles and surgery.

AMAZING ISN'T IT?

THE MYTH OR THE TRUTH?

The choice is yours to believe whatever you wish.
Here's the myth:
Straight Chiropractors are back doctors.

Here's the truth:
Straight Chiropractors are not "back doctors". However, they do work directly with the spine, which lies within the region of the back.

Chiropractic is the science, art and philosophy which utilizes the inherent recuperative powers of the body and deals with the relationship between the spinal column and the nerve system, as well as the role of that relationship in the restoration and maintenance of proper human performance.

Straight Chiropractors correct vertebral subluxations which occur through much of life's stressful traumas such as: birth, slips and falls as a child and as an adult, auto accidents, sports injuries, work related accidents, and habits which are not conducive to healthy living.

Chiropractic is a non-duplicating science, art and philosophy, in that what Straight Chiropractors offer in the way of self improvement is unique and not available anywhere else. Chiropractic enables the body to make use of its free and abundant energy for a complete expression of its own innate potential, thus improving human performance at all levels of the human experience, including health (being 15% of the human experience).

AMAZING ISN'T IT?

IS THERE CHIROPRACTIC RESEARCH?

Advances in medical science and the wonders of modern technology have removed a lot of mystery and risk formerly associated with childbirth. Few people realize, however, that the birth process is now being recognized as one of the foremost causes of vertebral subluxations. Even during normal uncomplicated infant deliveries, the spine is subject to extreme pressure from contractions and pushing as well as severe traction on the neck from pulling. New studies are revealing that spinal degeneration and distortions in the young and elderly were probably present as young as infancy and are often due to the birth process itself. These first subluxations, if left uncorrected, can result in irreversible nerve damage. Nerve interference and irritation from cervical spine (or neck) trauma at birth are known to cause abnormal function, unusual behavior and sometimes, in extreme cases, death.

Abraham Towbin, MD, is a neuropathologist at Harvard Medical School. He is one of many world authorities investigating the relationship between the birth process and spinal damage. He found that one of every three "stillborn" infants examined appeared to have actually died of cervical injuries during childbirth. In one of his many published articles Dr. Towbin states: "during the last part of delivery, during the final extraction of the fetus, mechanical stress imposed by obstetrical manipulation, even the application of standard orthodox procedures, may be intolerable to the fetus". Chiropractors have long advocated that children should have their spines examined as early as possible after birth. "As the twig bends, so grows the tree" is an old adage that is so appropriate when dealing with the development of the human spine.

Unlike the offspring of most other mammals, it takes several months of development before a human baby's muscles are strong enough to hold the head erect. The various stages of development witness the usual progression from head elevation and rotation to crawling, walking and running. Although we usually overlook incidents of a child falling, twisting or bumping during this formative period, evidence now shows us that these early months are critical to the formation of a healthy spine and nervous system. It is during these vulnerable stages that we should begin to concern ourselves with a child's spinal health. Chiropractors are fast becoming primary health care providers to many families because they understand that the spinal column is subject to early trauma through otherwise normal incidents in the early life of a child.

Not surprisingly, chiropractic care for children of all ages is rapidly gaining in popularity. We are witnessing a revolution in people's attitude toward their health and that of their young. Because chiropractic specializes in the detection of possible nerve damage resulting from vertebral subluxations, it is common today to witness an entire family going to the chiropractor for a spinal examination.

The spine is the "lifeline of the body" and must be protected at all times to ensure the healthiest possible future.

AMAZING ISN'T IT?

PRO-CHIROPRACTIC OR ANTI-CHIROPRACTIC?

Surf the internet and read through the pages of Time to review some great historical ideas and you will find a recurrent pattern. Time and time again, major breakthroughs in society's development have been met with tremendous opposition. Repeatedly, people's insistence on being "creatures of habit" has served only to prolong an attitude of stubbornness and prevent the benefits to be had by meeting and understanding a **NEW** idea. Let's face it, we hate the **NEW** because it causes us to feel uncomfortable as we are called to take a risk to do something we are unfamiliar with and will require us to change our inner center of gravity. In other words: to change our beliefs.

The key is to be open-minded, a quality the explorer Columbus found hard to come by when he suggested that the world was round. Galileo was excommunicated for having seen the earth revolving around the sun and it took several hundred years of factual data for the Pope to confess that the Church had been wrong and ask God and the world pardon for its awful transgression. Franklin, Edison, Marconi, the Wright Brothers, Einstein and now Steven Hawkins yearned for the public to have an open mind but people laughed at the notion of electricity, scorned the concept of wire-less sound, dismissed as absurd the possibility of men and women being able to fly, never believed atomic energy until the tragedy of the H-bomb and today refuse to deal with the fact that time and space do not exist as such and that it is a byproduct of man's illusion. Still, despite a general unwillingness to allow for an innovative concept, these pioneers in research and technology and numerous others like them persisted and continue to persist in the value and rewards of their ideas.

Today, Straight Chiropractors present yet another **"NEW"** discovery which concerns human performance. It has been opposed since 1895 and continues to meet adverse press from those who will not or do not take the time to research the merits of the Chiropractic Philosophy. It is based on a principle so beautiful in its simplicity that it seems a radical change to each of our established thoughts and concepts. Stated simply, Straight Chiropractors recognize that there is an inborn intelligence that created and organized you from two tiny cells, which gave you life and maintains it. Straight Chiropractors realize that health has nothing to do with symptoms or diseases and makes up only 15% of the human experience. Lack of health is caused by a body not functioning properly. It is simply common sense that if your body is working right, you're healthy; if your body is not working properly, you're lacking health! Correct the cause of the malfunction, and you restore the body to its natural, harmonious state of health.

Chiropractic flourishes not only because it makes good sense, but also because it works! This **"NEW IDEA"** recognizes that the greatest healer of all time was neither Hippocrates, the Father of Medicine, nor David Daniel Palmer, the discoverer of chiropractic. The greatest healer of all time is the innate intelligence within you! This innate intelligence is the sustaining life principle within each and every organism on our planet. This innate intelligence is responsible for the creation of NEW cells within the human body during every moment of its existence. Healing is the action of normal cells' replacement within the human body taking over the abnormal cells which have been produced as a result of a malfunction within the body interfering with this innate intelligence of life.

Let's look at this process more deeply. All body functions are directed by the innate intelligence of the body using the brain as master coordinator through the nerve system. The innate intelligence of the body uses the nerve system to freely control all defense mechanisms and healing processes through cellular replication. The job of the Straight Chiropractor is vital and direct by dealing with the spine which houses and protects the central nerve system. By keeping the 24 movable segments of the spine in proper position, the Straight Chiropractor insures a proper nerve supply to each cell, therefore assuring normal cell replacement which in turn becomes a proper functioning body. The result is a better expression of the innate intelligence of the body which gives rise to an improvement of human performance, thereby bringing about more health.

This **"NEW METHOD"** is so simple that it had been fought and resisted by the medical establishment for over 100 years much in the same way that Franklin, Edison, Einstein, Hawkins and Palmer discovered something **NEW.** And, believe it or not, that's how human beings react to the **NEW.**

AMAZING ISN'T IT?

ARE YOU LOOKING FOR HEALTH THROUGH A KEYHOLE?

For centuries man has been looking for health through the keyhole of therapy (treating effects): "No symptoms? I'm okay." Why then, the "sudden" heart attack, the "sudden" gall bladder attack, the "sudden" kidney stones, the "sudden" cancer? No warning! No pain, no symptoms, nothing out of the ordinary and "bam!" All of a "sudden"? You've got to be kidding! As most of you know, there is no such thing as "sudden" when it comes to the human body. It takes time to get to that point (9 months to create a baby, 90 days to replace heart cells, 120 for red blood cells, 12 years for puberty, 4 months for the first tooth, 5 days for stomach lining cells, etc.). Cardiologists say it takes about 8-10 years of heart malfunction for cardiac problems to show up as symptoms. Nephrologists say it takes 6-7 years of kidney malfunction for kidney problems to show up as symptoms. Oncologists say it takes sometimes 20-30 years for certain body parts to malfunction for cancer to show up as symptoms. Indeed, there is no process that does not require time.

So we begin to realize that symptoms don't tell the tale. Chiropractic, which is not a treatment of symptoms and diseases, is the unique art, science and philosophy that recognizes one common element in all body malfunctions.

When the body does not function properly, it does not heal properly, it does not have the proper resistance to defend itself against viruses, germs and bacteria and most important of all, it does not live properly. Straight Chiropractors recognize that malfunction of the body occurs when there is an interference to the nerve energy flow from brain cells to tissue cells or from tissue cells to brain cells within the nerve system caused by vertebral subluxations.

Stated differently, a vertebral subluxation is an insult to the nerve system caused by a slight pressure of a vertebra on the spinal cord and nerves. The end result of a vertebral subluxation is a lack of proper transmission of mental impulses (which is nerve energy) from the brain to the parts of the body to malfunction. Of course, basic science textbooks agree that the central nerve system (brain and spinal cord) is the major organ of communication within the human body. Yet, somehow this fact does not get much beyond the cobwebs of those pages.

In Columbus' time they believed the earth was flat and if anyone ventured near the edge... well... goodbye Charlie! But old Chris Columbus had the courage to sail across the Atlantic and found a NEW world in the process. We feel sure there were many in Queen Isabella's court who called him "radical" or "fanatic". They were the ones who based their opinion on "authority", when in fact, it was based on fear of the unknown, of basically losing what they knew and felt secure with and therefore they were ignorant of the truth of the matter. They put Galileo in jail for daring to suggest that the earth revolved around the sun and not vice-versa. The "authorities" put D.D. Palmer, the discoverer of Chiropractic, in jail too, because he had the courage to speak out about a whole NEW approach to understanding how the human body works. Now, Straight Chiropractors know, beyond any doubt, what's out there: the body revolves around the nerve system just as the earth revolves around the sun. This is an immutable law. Science is finally catching up with Straight Chiropractors and recognizes this supreme truth. Don't be caught in the "flat world" of thinking.

Health is not the presence or absence of symptoms. Health is whether the life-energy gets from the brain to the 70 trillion cells of your body in the normal quantity and quality. The vertebra can put pressure on the nerve system and interfere with that life-energy. If we are ever to reach our God-given birthright of healthy life without fear, then let's make sure we get our spine checked weekly for the detection and correction of vertebral subluxations.

Next time you hear "fanatic" or "radical", in regards to Straight Chiropractors, remember how people thought the earth was flat and how the solar system revolved around it. Straight Chiropractors are ahead of their time, like Columbus and Galileo.

AMAZING ISN'T IT?

CURRICULUM VITAE
DR. CLAUDE LESSARD

B.S. Limestone College, Gaffney, S.C.   1977

Doctor Of Chiropractic Degree, Sherman College Of Chiropractic,
Spartanburg, S.C.   1977

Internship, Sherman College Of Chiropractic   1977

Recipient Of The B.J. Palmer Chiropractic Philosophy Distinction Award, S.C.C.   1977

Recipient Of The B.J. Palmer Clinical Excellence Award, S.C.C.   1977

Diplomate Of The National Board Of Chiropractic Examiner

Certificated Of Preliminary Professional Education #C35301,
Commonwealth Of Pennsylvania

Commonwealth Of Pa License #DC-1702-L

Co-Founder And Charter Member Of Adio Institute Of Straight Chiropractic   1978

Assistant Professor Of Chiropractic Philosophy, Adio I.S.C.   1978-80

Student Referral Counselor, Adio I.S.C.   1978-81

Administrative Dean Of College Adio I.S.C.   1979-80

Associate Professor Of Chiropractic Technique, Adio I.S.C.   1980-81

Director Of Community Health Center, Adio I.S.C.   1980-81

Member Of Chiropractic Life Fellowship Of PA

Member Of F.S.C.O. (Federation Of Straight Chiropractors Organizations)

Graduate Of Church Ministry Program, St. Charles Borromeo Seminary   1983-87

Certified Myotech Examiner

Chiropractor Of The Month Award, Markson Management Service,   1988

Chiropractor Of The Year Award, Markson Management Services   1992

Postgraduate Course Of Study In Applied Spinal Biomechanics From
The Aragona Spinal Biomechanic Engineering Laboratory, Incorporated   1992

Member Of Distinguished Board Of Regent, Sherman College   Since 1993

Chiropractor Of The Year Award, Quest Management Systems   1993

Member Of Parker Chiropractic Resources Foundation

Chair And Co-Author Of Audio Book
"Spirit Of '76" Sherman College Of Chiropractic   1996

Founder Of C.A.C.E. (Clients Association For Chiropractic Education)   1997

Licensed Private Pilot Single Engine Airplanes Land   1998

Founder Of Lessard Institute For Chiropractic Clients   1998

Recipient Of The Spirit Of Sherman College Of Chiropractic Award   1999

Licensed Instrument Airplanes   2000

Author Of Book "Chiropractic Amazing Isn't It?"   2003

Chiropractor Of The Year Award, Sherman College Of Chiropractic   2006

Resolution 5553-09-06 Extrait Des Proces-Verbeaux
Ville De Sainte-Anne De Beaupre   2006

Author Of Book "Quiropraxia No Es Asombrosa?"   2010

Author Of Book "La Chiropratique, Incroyable N'est-Ce Pas?"   2012

Author Of Blue Book "A New Look At Chiropractic Basic Science"   2017

Author Of Blue Book "Una Mirada A La Sciencia Básica Quiropráctia"   2019

Author Of Book "Chiropractic Amazing Isn't It?" Workbook   2020

Author Of Book "Quiropraxia ¿No Es Asombrosa?" Manual De Trabaja   2020

RESOURCES

Sherman College of Chiropractic
2020 Springfield Road
P.O. Box 1452
Spartanburg, S.C. 29304

Federation of Straight Chiropractors Organizations
642 Broad Street
Clifton, NJ 07013
1-800-521-9856

Foundation for the Advancement of Chiropractic Education
P.O. Box 1052
Levittown, PA 19058
1-800-397-9722

Clients Association for Chiropractic Education
210 Makefield Road
Morrisville, PA 19067
1-215-736-8816